Producing Patient Information

HOW TO RESEARCH, DEVELOP AND PRODUCE
EFFECTIVE INFORMATION RESOURCES

The King's Fund is an independent charitable foundation working for better health, especially in London. We carry out research, policy analysis and development activities, working on our own, in partnerships, and through grants. We are a major resource to people working in health, offering leadership and education courses; seminars and workshops; publications; information and library services; and conference and meeting facilities.

Published by:
King's Fund
11–13 Cavendish Square
London W1G 0AN
www.kingsfund.org.uk

© King's Fund 2003

Charity registration number: 207401

First published as *The POPPi Guide*, 2000

ISBN 1 85717 470 4

A CIP catalogue record for this book is available from the British Library.

Available from:
King's Fund
11–13 Cavendish Square
London W1G 0AN
Tel: 020 7307 2591
Fax: 020 7307 2801
www.kingsfundbookshop.org.uk

Edited by Eleanor Stanley and Sonia Shepherd
Cover design by Minuche Mazumdar Farrar
Cover photo from Getty Images
Typeset by Grasshopper Design Company
Printed and bound in Great Britain

Outline

Focusing primarily on the NHS in England and Wales, this section briefly outlines ways in which health sector organisations are incorporating public involvement into their ways of working. It highlights key policy developments and other initiatives that are pertinent to producers of patient information.

The section will be of most use to those wishing to gain a policy context to patient information production, and to those looking for 'hooks' upon which to support funding or similar applications.

It is always tempting to jump straight in and start doing something. This section suggests pausing to consider why your organisation wishes to produce patient information. If this is not already clear, it will help you determine how the production of patient information fits in with your organisation's overarching information policy. Different types of organisation will need policies with different emphases. The section then points to some broader issues that you will need to consider initially, and indeed later on in the development process, such as legal liability.

Why do you want to produce information, who is it for and where can you find information that may already exist? These are some of the topics discussed in the first half of this section. The second half looks at project planning – timescales, teamwork, budgets and the like – and introduces the need for early thinking about dissemination.

Section 8 Dissemination

This section presents some ways to get your resources known about – if that is what you want. Depending upon your organisational set up, this may be something that is taken care of by people in other departments, for example, in marketing or communications. Even if that is the case, it will be useful to read this section, both for additional ideas and because you will need to consider dissemination when you plan how many copies you will produce. It is also important for you to have thought through not only the production issues, but also how to make sure your material reaches the right place and the right people.

Section 9 Evaluating and updating

People do not buy food that is past its sell by date, so why should they accept information that is not current? It is just as dangerous – if not more so. This section considers when and how to review your information on a regular basis and takes a brief tour of the ways you may want to more formally evaluate your product once it has been developed and distributed.

Contents

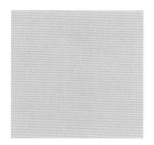

Figures

Foreword

The Government and the health service are strongly committed to involving users. They are working hard to put the patient and the public at the centre of a modernised NHS.

Provision of information is the platform upon which this empowerment and partnership are built. The NHS Plan outlines an array of ways in which the health service wishes to involve and inform patients. From Patient Advice and Liaison Services to a range of NHS Direct initiatives, the NHS is meeting its promise to provide members of the public with information they can access and understand.

Quality of information is paramount. By establishing and providing continued support for the Centre for Health Information Quality, and through the current NHS Identity work on improving the presentation of patient information, the NHS has made a commitment to providing the highest quality resources.

It is with this theme in mind that I welcome *Producing Patient Information*, which provides thorough and practical insights for those wishing to excel in the production of health resources, whether they work within the NHS and its allied professions, or in the voluntary or commercial sectors.

Lord Hunt of King's Heath OBE
Parliamentary Under Secretary, Department of Health

About the author

A pharmacist by profession, Mark Duman gained extensive experience in health communications during his involvement in a number of patient information projects at Health Care International, Lewisham Hospital NHS Trust, the King's Fund, the BBC and Hutchison Whampoa. He founded the Patient Information Forum, the pecmi Working Group and the Ask About Medicines Week initiative, and today works as an independent health care communications consultant. He has lectured and written extensively on health information issues and is a judge for the BMA Patient Information and BUPA Foundation Communication Awards.

Acknowledgements

In addition to those people who helped with the first edition, a number of people have been important in helping revise this guide.

- Vikki Enwistle, Programme Director (Participation in Health Care), Health Services Research Unit, University of Aberdeen; Mary Last of the Patient Information Forum, who set up the BMA's patient information award, and Jane Shaddock, Project Manager, Centre for Health Information Quality for their insightful reviews of the revised edition
- Helen Crisp and Sasha Shepherd for their respective updates to information on HQS and DISCERN
- David Gilbert from the Commission for Health Improvement who kindly reviewed the Patient and Public Involvement section
- Julie Glanville, Associate Director, NHS Centre for Review and Dissemination; Information Service Manager, NHS CRD/Centre for Health Economics University of York, for her comments on the section on clinical evidence
- Lynne Jones at Colon Cancer Concern for sharing her expertise in putting patient information on the internet
- Sarah Ransome at the Blood Pressure Association for providing an excellent case study on using patient feedback to update materials, and indeed to all those who kindly provided case study material
- The Centre for Health information Quality (CHIQ) for again agreeing to receive the feedback form (at the back of this guide)
- Fiona McLean at the British Library for her outstanding contributions to the bibliography and further reading sections
- Caroline Miller at the Chartered Society of Physiotherapy Library for pointing out some additional sources of consumer health information
- Christine Farrell for her support and guidance in writing the first edition and her encouragement in revising the second
- The King's Fund publishing team for suggesting and supporting a revised edition
- Tanya, Malka and Yonah Duman for their patience and understanding in allowing me to use some of our precious family time to conduct this revision, and of course to HaShem.

Mark Duman

Definitions and acronyms

Who is a 'patient'?

The term 'patient' is in common use in the National Health Service (NHS) and, while we understand that not everyone approves of the passive concept associated with this word, we have used it throughout in the knowledge that it is widely understood. We use it in this guide to refer to all health-service users, including individuals with specific disease states, their carers, and people seeking information on health promotion and disease prevention.

What is 'patient information'?

The term 'patient information' refers to information that is produced and provided, in any medium, for the benefit of patients (see the definition above). This could include information on specific disease states (such as diabetes or arthritis), on health services (such as going into hospital or entering a clinical trial) and on health promotion issues (such as smoking cessation or healthy eating).

Other terms commonly used for this purpose include 'consumer health information', 'health information', 'health promotion' and 'patient education materials'. We do not use 'patient information' here to refer to patient identifiable data, such as that contained within medical records.

Acronyms

ABTI	Association of the British Pharmaceutical Industry
AIOPI	Association of Information Officers in the Pharmaceutical Industry
BMA	British Medical Association
BMJ	British Medical Journal
BNF	British National Formulary
BSL	British Sign Language
CASP	Critical Appraisal Skills Programme
CIS	Cancer Information Strategy
CHIC	Consumer Health Information Consortium
CHIQ	Centre for Health Information Quality
CNST	Clinical Negligence Scheme for Trusts
COREC	Central Office of Research Ethics Committees
DDA	Disability Discrimination Act 1995
DISCERN	Developing an Assessment Instrument for the Clinical Appraisal of Written Consumer Health Information
EQIP	Ensuring Quality Information for Patients
ERG	external reference group
HCI	Health Coalition Initiative
HDA	Health Development Agency
HEA	Health Education Authority
HEBS	Health Education Board for Scotland

HQS	Health Quality Service
NeLH	National electronic Library for Health
NHS	National Health Service
NHSCRD	NHS Centre for Reviews and Dissemination
NHSDO	NHS Direct Online
NHSIA	NHS Information Authority
NICE	National Institute for Clinical Evidence
NSF	National Service Framework
PAGB	Proprietary Association of Great Britain
PALS	Patient Advisory and Liaison Service
PCT	primary care trust
pecmi	Promoting Excellence in Consumer Medicines Information
PiF	Patient information Forum
PIL	patient information leaflet
POPPi	Practicalities of Producing Patient information
PPC	Promoting Patient Choice
RCCM	Research Council on Complementary Medicines
RCT	randomised controlled trial
RF	readability factor
RNIB	Royal National Institute of the Blind
RNID	Royal National Institute for Deaf People
SIGN	Scottish Intercollegiate Guidelines Network
TriLET	Trials Leaflet Evaluation Tool

Introduction

Who is this guide for?

Producing Patient Information: How to research, develop and produce effective information resources is for people who want to produce and provide health information. It is the second edition of *The POPPi Guide*, published by the King's Fund in 2000. It is intended primarily for people working in the NHS – in hospital settings and in primary care – but it will also be useful for voluntary organisations and university departments specialising in health care, for pharmaceutical companies and for health communications agencies.

Its main aim is excellence in the production of health resources. We know that it may not always be possible to achieve the 'gold standard' of production outlined in this guide, but working towards high standards is an important part of the process.

However, producing information is only one part of the overall picture. There is little point in producing great information that sits on shelves. Close consideration needs to be given to ways of disseminating the information once it has been produced, and in ensuring feedback is gathered on the usefulness of the product.

How to use the guide

The guide has been written as a hands-on resource to meet the needs of readers with different requirements.

Readers who are new to the field of patient information production will find it useful to read the guide from cover to cover. The first section provides background information on the need for patient information and links this into government initiatives. Subsequent sections then take the reader through the process of producing information, step by step. Sections 8 and 9 look at ways of disseminating, evaluating and updating the information.

Readers with more experience of producing patient information may prefer to dip in and out of the resource to gain additional insights into topics of particular interest.

Whatever your level of experience, the guide uses the following elements to help you:

- section overviews, which summarise each section and provide signposts on who should read what
- action points, which sum up each section at a glance
- case studies and illustrations from information packages, offering an opportunity to learn from other people's experience
- information points for additional useful details
- further reading sections at relevant points throughout the book.

1 PROCESS MAP

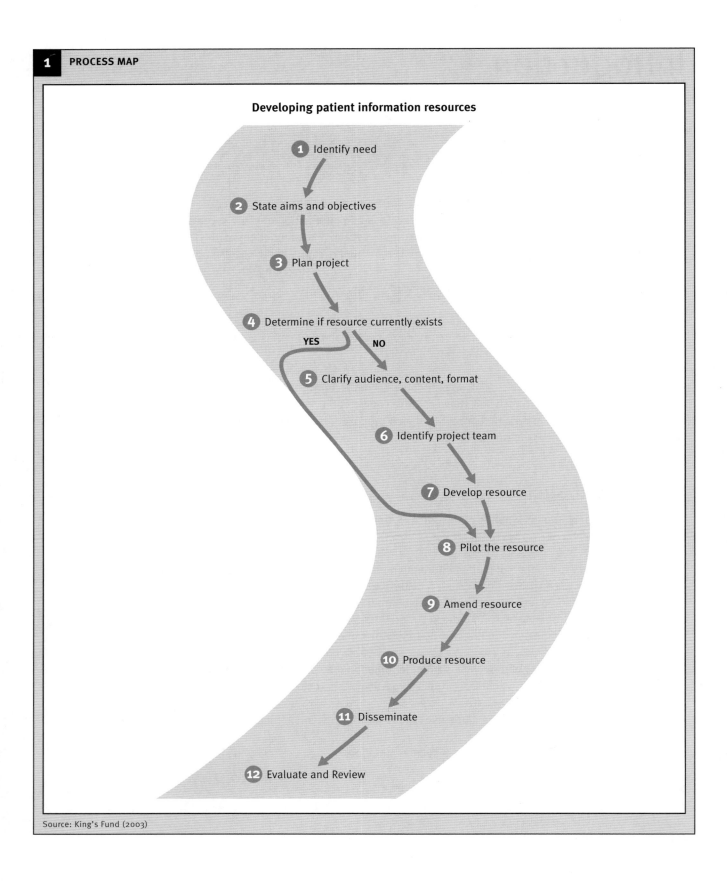

Developing patient information resources

1. Identify need
2. State aims and objectives
3. Plan project
4. Determine if resource currently exists
   - YES
   - NO
5. Clarify audience, content, format
6. Identify project team
7. Develop resource
8. Pilot the resource
9. Amend resource
10. Produce resource
11. Disseminate
12. Evaluate and Review

Source: King's Fund (2003)

The guide cannot answer every question about producing health information, so an extensive listings section at the back of the book contains sources of specialist information for people who need more technical help, including:

- contact details for all organisations mentioned in the guide
- information about funding sources
- useful websites
- references for further reading and a bibliography.

Finally, as the reader, your feedback is very valuable to us, so we have included a feedback form to enable us to determine what you would consider useful to future editions.

Further reading

The following books and literature reviews provide excellent background to the topics of informed choice and consumer health information:

British Medical Journal, 18 September 1999 (*BMJ*, vol 319, issue 7212). An entire issue dedicated to the development of partnership between doctors and patients. Another patient-themed issue is planned for June 2003.

Coulter A (2002). *The Autonomous Patient: Ending paternalism in medical care*. London: Nuffield Trust/TSO. Reviews how patients can play a more active role, including their information needs.

Coulter A, Magee H (in press). *The European Patient of the Future*. Buckingham: Open University Press. Describes a study conducted in eight European countries on patients' views on communication with health care professionals, options for accessing health advice (including the internet and telemedicine), their information needs and attitudes to involvement, choice and patients' rights.

Edwards A, Elwyn G eds (2001). *Evidence-based Patient Choice – Inevitable or impossible?* Oxford: Oxford University Press. Provides a collection of research, clinical examples and patient narratives on this topic.

Entwistle V, O'Donnell M (1999). *A Guide to Producing Health Information*. Aberdeen: Aberdeen University. An online guide to producing health information including an excellent section on information needs and gaps in research evidence @ www.abdn.ac.uk/hsru/guide.hti

Garlick W (2003). *Patient Information – What's the prognosis?* London: Consumers Association. A wide-ranging report on the provision in the UK of information about medicines, therapies and illnesses.

Gray M, Rutter H (2002). *The Resourceful Patient*. Oxford: eRosetta. A web-based book and toolkit for those seeking to address the problems of health care in the 21st century. Available at: www.resourcefulpatient.org

Olszewski D, Jones L (1998). *Putting People in the Picture*. Edinburgh, Scottish Association of Health Councils. Reviews the literature on information for patients and the public about illness and treatment.

MacDougall J (1998). *Well Read: Developing consumer health information in Ireland*. Wexford: Library Association of Ireland. Considers the fast-growing area of consumer health information and makes a number of recommendations.

Although not the focus of this guide, it is important to mention that producing and providing good quality, evidence-based patient information must complement – not replace – communication with health care professionals. The *British Medical Journal's* theme issue of 28 September 2002 discusses some of these communication challenges.

Two other publications aim to help patients obtain a better understanding of the system in which health care is delivered:

Hammond P, Mosley M (2000). *Trust Me I'm a Doctor*. London: Metro Books. Gives patients encouragement and information to move from blind trust to informed scepticism. It examines health issues from a consumer's perspective, exposing myths and highlighting the gap between scientific evidence and treatment.

Harvey S, Wylie I (1999). *Patient Power: Getting the best from your healthcare*. New York: Simon and Schuster.

Guide →

1 Why provide information?

Focusing primarily on the NHS in England and Wales, this section briefly outlines ways in which health sector organisations are incorporating public involvement into their ways of working. It highlights key policy developments and other initiatives that are pertinent to producers of patient information.

The section will be of most use to those wishing to gain a policy context to patient information production, and to those looking for 'hooks' upon which to support funding or similar applications.

Most, if not all, of the readers of this publication will already be convinced of the need to provide patients with high quality information. However, some of the people you interact with – other health care professionals or management – may be less convinced that this is a worthwhile use of often scarce resources. Although much research still needs to be done, there is increasing evidence that providing high quality patient information is beneficial to patients, health care professionals and health care providers.

REASONS FOR PROVIDING PATIENTS WITH INFORMATION

- *to understand what is wrong*
- *to gain a realistic idea of prognosis*
- *to make the most of consultations*
- *to understand the process and likely outcomes of possible tests and treatments*
- *to assist in self-care*
- *to provide reassurance and help to cope*
- *to help others understand*
- *to legitimise help-seeking and concerns*
- *to identify further information and self-help groups*
- *to identify the 'best' health-care providers.*

Source: Coulter A, Entwistle V, Gilbert D (1998). *Informing Patients*. London: King's Fund.

Further reading

England PA (1999). 'Patient information'. *Journal of Audiovisual Media in Medicine*, vol 22, pp 7–14. This discusses the benefits of providing patients with information, against a background of political history, legal requirements and the element of design, including recommendations for improving quality.

Kirkham M, Stapleton H eds (2001). *Informed Choice in Maternity Care: An evaluation of evidence based leaflets*. University of York: NHS Centre for Reviews and Dissemination.

NHS Centre for Reviews and Dissemination (2000). 'Informing, communicating and sharing decisions with people who have cancer'. *Effective Health Care Bulletin*, vol 6(6).

O'Connor AM, Rostom A, Fiset V, Tetroe J, Entwistle V, Llewellyn-Thomas H, Holmes-Rovner M, Barry M, Jones J (2002). 'Decision aids for people facing health treatment or screening decisions: systematic review'. *BMJ*, vol 319, pp 731–4.

Key policy developments

Numerous changes have taken place in the NHS on the topic of public involvement – and specifically in that of patient information – since the first edition of this guide was published in March 2000.

The majority of NHS bodies in England, both new and old, have a mandate through the NHS Plan to involve the public and patients in the way they operate. New positions – often called 'Head/Director of Patient and Public Involvement' – can be found at the Department of Health, Commission for Health Improvement, the Audit Commission and the National Patient Safety Agency, to name but a few. For those interested in the topic of patient and public involvement, a list of further reading references is provided on the previous page.

The NHS Information Authority (NHSIA) has established the Public Reference Group, a database of nearly 500 patients, carers and citizens willing to provide input and help the authority improve existing resources and services and develop new ones. The National Institute for Clinical Excellence (NICE) has recruited the public to a Citizen's Council to enable NICE to reflect public opinion in the guidance it publishes on the clinical and cost effectiveness of treatments and care for the NHS. Many of the royal colleges have patient liaison groups, and even such an august academic body as the Medical Research Council now has a consumer liaison group.

The Government is introducing a new system for involving patients and the public in health that will take over from Community Health Councils. This system will include the new Commission for Patient and Public Involvement in Health, patients' forums in all trusts and a service for providing independent support and advice to complainants through the Patients Advice and Liaison Service (PALS).

The NHS Plan

@
www.nhs.uk/nationalplan

The NHS Plan has patient and public involvement at its core. Patient information is quoted as the second of the NHS's core principles and focuses on the provision of 'information services and support to individuals in relation to health promotion, disease prevention, self-care, rehabilitation and after care' (Department of Health 2002a, p 3). Chapter 10 of the NHS Plan, entitled 'Changes for patients', covers this topic and states that referral letters will regularly be copied to patients and that better information will help patients choose a GP. It also outlines the services to be provided by NHS Direct through a wide array of channels, from telephones and websites to touch-screen kiosks and interactive digital TV.

@
The NHS Guide is available at: www.nhs.uk/nhsguide
The official gateway to National Health Service organisations on the internet can be found at: www.nhs.uk

The NHS Plan, attempting to practice what it preaches, also produced a 'patient-friendly' version of the points most pertinent to patients: *The NHS Guide*. This supercedes the Patient's Charter.

Patient Advice and Liaison Services

www.doh.gov.uk/patient
adviceandliaisonservices/
dohpalstandards.pdf

PALS is central to the new system of patient and public involvement introduced in the NHS Plan in 2000. It does not replace specialist advocacy services such as mental health and learning disability but will be complementary to existing services. All NHS trusts and primary care trusts were expected to establish a PALS by April 2002. One of their core responsibilities, as quoted in Department of Health guidance issued in Jan 2002, is to 'provide accurate information to patients, families and carers, about the Trust's services and other health related issues, using accredited reliable sources' (Department of Health 2002b, p 9).

www.moorfields.co.uk/
ForPatients/PALS

The Moorfields Eye Hospital NHS Trust website promoted its PALS as offering the following:

- to help answer your questions about your care
- to advise and support you and your family. We understand that being unwell can be an anxious time and you might need someone else to liase on your behalf
- to guide you and your family, relative or friend through the different services available
- to respond to any concerns you may have about your care
- to provide an information centre for advice and support on health and care issues related to your condition
- to listen to your suggestions.

Other policy initiatives

Patient information may be linked to national and local policy initiatives such as those outlined below:

Toolkit for Producing Patient Information

The Department of Health has a programme of work in the context of the 'patient experience' agenda to improve patient information across the NHS. The NHS Plan commitment to putting patients at the centre of care lays some firm foundations for giving patients more power, protection and choices. The Department of Health has developed written guidance and supportive templates to make it easier for the NHS to produce good quality information that meets the needs of patients and the public, in addition to its own needs. The guidance was put together with the help of:

The *Toolkit for Producing Patient Information* is available on the NHS Identity website at www. doh.gov.uk/nhsidentity. Hard copies can be obtained from the NHS Responseline on 0870 155 5455, quoting reference number 29682

- the Patient Information Forum, a national group representing people working in the field of patient information in the NHS and the voluntary sector
- the Royal National Institute of the Blind
- the Plain English Campaign.

See Presentation (p 54), which includes extracts from the toolkit.

The Expert Patient

www.doh.gov.uk/cmo/
ep-report.pdf

The Expert Patient initiative – 'a new approach to chronic disease management for the 21st century' – recognises and funds work around the fact that in some cases, patients with chronic conditions know their diseases better than some health care professionals. The programme, started in August 2001, brings together patient groups, academics and health care professionals to look at ways in which patients with chronic disease can participate in lay-led self-management programmes around their own conditions.

@
www.doh.gov.uk/cancer/
cis.htm

Cancer Information Strategy

The Cancer Information Strategy (CIS) can be viewed as the outcome of a number of policy initiatives, including the NHS Cancer Plan, NHS Information Strategy and National Service Framework (NSF) work (*see opposite*). It forms one of five such information strategies to support NSF topics and seems the most advanced in its patient information work. From this perspective, it:

- aims to ensure that accurate, comprehensive and comprehensible information about cancer is accessible to all those who need it
- seeks to enhance the quality of care given to patients with actual or suspected cancer, by ensuring that their needs for information are met in a timely, sensitive and appropriate way, and by ensuring good communication between health care sectors
- provides a useful breakdown of information needs according to the perspectives of different users and the need for different types of subjects of information.

Patient Partnership Strategy

This UK NHS initiative was launched in 1996. The aims of the strategy included:

- supporting users of NHS services and their carers in gaining a greater voice and influence as active partners with professionals
- enabling patients to become informed about their treatment and care, and to be able to make informed decisions and choices about it if they wish.

In autumn 1999, the Department of Health launched a revised version of its 1996 strategy. Entitled *Patient and Public Involvement in the New NHS* (Department of Health 1999a), which restates the importance of partnerships between the NHS and the public, gives examples of national and local initiatives in partnership developments and identifies future action to be taken.

@
www.nhsia.nhs.uk/def/
pages/info4health/5.asp

Information for Health

Information for Health, issued in September 1998, outlines an information strategy for the modern NHS between 1998 and 2005. The strategy aims:

- to make sure NHS professionals have the information they need to provide care and to play their part in improving the public's health
- to ensure that patients, carers and the public have the information they need to make decisions about their own treatment and care
- to influence the shape of health services generally.

Chapter 5 of the strategy focuses on meeting public and patient needs and supports the concept of shared decision-making, by aiming to:

- eliminate unnecessary travel and delay for patients, by providing remote online access to services, specialists and care wherever practicable
- provide access for NHS patients to accredited, independent multimedia background information and advice about their condition
- provide fast, convenient access for the public to accredited multimedia advice on lifestyle and health, and information to support public involvement in – and understanding of – local and NHS policy development.

The strategy also discusses the role of the Centre for Health Information Quality (CHIQ, *see* p 87) in working with producers of information to improve its quality, accessibility and evidence base.

Building the Information Core: Implementing the NHS Plan

@ www.nhsia.nhs.uk/def/ pages/info_core/overview. asp (sample pages)

This strategy was published in January 2001 as an update to *Information for Health*. It outlines the necessary information and IT infrastructure investment required to deliver the NHS Plan and support patient-centred care and services. Chapter 4 focuses on information services such as NHS Direct.

Bristol Enquiry

@ www.doh.gov.uk/ bristolinquiryresponse/ bristolresponsech8.htm

The importance of patient information has also been mentioned in the Department of Health's Response to the Bristol Royal Infirmary Public Enquiry.

National Service Frameworks

@ www.doh.gov.uk/nsf

National Service Frameworks (NSF) were launched in April 1998 to establish sets of national standards and define service models for a series of defined services-of-care groups. Each NSF is developed with the assistance of an external reference group (ERG) that brings together health care professionals, service users and carers, health service managers, partner agencies and other advocates. ERGs adopt an inclusive process to engage the full range of views. The Department of Health supports the ERGs and manages the overall process.

Each framework will include statements about seeking information from patients and carers to ensure that the NHS is sensitive to individual needs. Every trust, including primary care trusts, will set and monitor standards for the way in which patients and their carers view the quality of the treatment and care they receive. These standards will include information and choice.

Securing Our Future Health: Taking a long-term view (Wanless Report)

@ www.hm-treasury.gov.uk/ mediastore/otherfiles/ chap 7.pdf (go to p 4)

An independent review by Derek Wanless, published in April 2002, is the first ever evidence-based assessment of the long-term resource requirements for the NHS. Chapter 7 summaries its conclusions and recommendations, one of which includes 'the development of improved health information to help people engage with their care in an informed way'.

See Informed consent and Confidentiality and use of patient data, p 16.

---

i

- To obtain copies of the Department of Health publications, call the NHS Responseline. Tel: 08701 0541 555 455 or email: doh@prolog.uk.com Most of their publications are also available free via the internet @ www.doh.gov.uk/publications/index.html
- There are links to official government documents from a range of departments @ www.official-document.co.uk
- Priced government publications are sold by the Stationery Office. Tel: 0870 600 5522 or email: book.orders@theso.co.uk

2 Before getting started

It is always tempting to jump straight in and start doing something. This section suggests pausing to consider why your organisation wishes to produce patient information. If this is not already clear, it will help you determine how the production of patient information fits in with your organisation's overarching information policy. Different types of organisation will need policies with different emphases. The section then points to some broader issues that you will need to consider initially, and indeed later on in the development process, such as legal liability.

Developing an information policy

Developing an information policy will involve many people, and should certainly include patients and their carers. Meeting their needs for information, as well as those of the organisation, should be a high priority. The production of specific information for patients will then fit into this policy. Section 1 sets the context for some of the main government policies and workstreams in the area of patient information.

Questions to ask

To develop an information policy, an agency or department needs to ask some questions:

- Is there, or should there be, a general corporate policy on information for patients?
- Who is responsible for policy, planning, providing information and setting priorities?
- Does the information policy cover the full range of topics and issues that concern patients and carers, and departments?
- Will there be a clear boundary between information and advice? All information services have to make this distinction, and it is important to be clear at the outset the exact purpose of all the information provided.
- Does the policy make it possible to meet new needs as they emerge?
- Does the policy allow for the use of all existing media and new media as they are developed?
- What resources are available for implementing the policy and who will be responsible for allocating and managing them?
- Who will have overall management responsibility for implementing, monitoring and reviewing the policy?

Corporate strategy and policy guidelines should include the roles and responsibilities for staff in charge of patient information. These responsibilities should include:

- deciding how patients are told about their rights
- providing access to records
- ensuring confidentiality
- setting up procedures for patients and carers who want to make positive comments or register complaints.

i

The Consumer Health Information Consortium (CHIC) is a support organisation for those interested in improving health information aimed at the public. It encourages good practice and promotes free and open access for all to health information (*see* Useful contacts, p 103).

The corporate information policy should also include issues such as the use of 'house style' to ensure that the presentation of printed material and the use of corporate logos are consistent. To promote consistent content, some organisations use a set of preferred terms and a common thesaurus.

Not only are organisations looking to promote consistency across their internal information functions, but in some cases there are moves to ensure national consistency. *See* the Department of Health *Toolkit for Producing Patient Information* (p 9).

Aims of the policy

Your organisation's information policy will be based on a general aim, which applies to all the information provided.

For example, in an NHS trust, one of the specific aims could be to ensure that patient information produced in-house:

- reflects what patients want to know and how they want to use it
- helps them receive the services to which they are entitled
- helps them understand their condition
- enables them to choose the treatment appropriate to their condition, if they so wish.

Another specific example is from within the pharmaceutical industry. Health care professionals are the main source of calls to medical information departments, but queries are also received from members of the general public. The Association of Information Officers in the Pharmaceutical Industry (AIOPI) convened a working party to create an industry standard for medical information functions. The AIOPI Guidelines (standards in medical information) were developed to provide a reference against which medical information departments can monitor and improve their performance in line with customer requirements.

@
www.aiopi.org.uk

Guidelines for patient information

If you work in an organisation in which the production of patient information is well established, you may feel it worthwhile to produce guidelines for use throughout the organisation. Ideally, a patient information officer or someone in the quality assurance department should take responsibility for producing guidelines and for making sure that they are used wherever information is produced. Once the guidelines have been agreed, they should be audited and updated regularly. The drive to improve patient information within NHS trusts can be linked with quality standards schemes (*see* p 82).

Some NHS trust hospitals have developed standards for producing patient information. These range from guidelines suggesting how material should be developed to protocols that require all patient resources to adhere to internal standards. Members of the Patient Information Forum have developed their own in-house guidance and share their experiences with each other (*see* Useful contacts, p 103).

→ **Action points**

- If you are considering developing guidelines for producing patient information, contact someone in your audit or quality assurance departments to discuss the best way to proceed.
- Get in touch with people in NHS trusts who may have produced guidelines to share experiences.
- Review and audit your guidelines regularly.

Case study: Developing standards

Richardson and Moran describe the process of developing standards for developing patient information in an NHS Trust:

> *The process... has been lengthy but has resulted in a cohesive and controlled approach to the production of patient information. Directorates still 'own' the process but are given support and assistance which was previously lacking. We are currently at the stage where the first leaflets are being produced which adhere to the standards. It will be necessary to evaluate the leaflets and standards, a process involving patients.*

Richardson and Moran (1995)

Further reading

Brighton Health Care NHS Trust (2001). *Guide to Producing Patient Information*. Brighton: Brighton Health Care NHS Trust.

Great Ormond Street Hospital for Children NHS Trust (2001). *How to Produce Information for Families*. London: Great Ormond Street Hospital for Children NHS Trust. Email: info@gosh.nhs.uk

Leicestershire and Rutland Healthcare NHS Trust (1999). *Step by Step Procedure for Developing a New Patient Information Leaflet*. Leicester: Leicestershire and Rutland Healthcare NHS Trust. Contact the Resources Department. Tel: 0116 258 8856

Mayday Healthcare NHS Trust (2002). *Policy for Producing Written Patient Information*. Croydon: Mayday Healthcare NHS Trust.

Nottingham City Hospital NHS Trust (1997). *Producing Written Information for Patients: Staff guidelines*. Nottingham: Nottingham City Hospital NHS Trust. Contact the communications manager. Tel: 0115 969 1169

Royal Berkshire and Battle Hospitals NHS Trust (1996). *Guidelines for Producing Written Information for Patients*. Reading: Royal Berkshire and Battle Hospitals NHS Trust. Tel: 01734 878 592

Sheffield Teaching Hospitals NHS Trust (2002). *Writing Information for Patients and the Public: Trust standards and guidelines*. Sheffield: Sheffield Teaching Hospitals NHS Trust. Contact the patient information officer. Tel: 0114 271 2243

Southern Derbyshire Acute Hospitals NHS Trust (June 2002a). *Out-patient Procedures Information Standards*. Derby: Southern Derbyshire Acute Hospitals NHS Trust.

Southern Derbyshire Acute Hospitals NHS Trust (June 2002b). *Procedure Specific Information Standards*. Derby: Southern Derbyshire Acute Hospitals NHS Trust.

Southern Derbyshire Acute Hospitals NHS Trust (June 2002c). *Specialty Specific Information Standards*. Derby: Southern Derbyshire Acute Hospitals NHS Trust.

Southern Derbyshire Acute Hospitals NHS Trust (June 2000d). *Patient Information Process*. Derby: Southern Derbyshire Acute Hospitals NHS Trust. Contact the patient information officer for all the above. Tel: 01332 347141

South Tyneside Primary Care Trust (2002). *Resource Production Protocol Summary*. Hebburn: South Tyneside Primary Care Trust.

Stockport Healthcare NHS Trust (1999). *Checklist of Trust Principles for Producing Written Information*. Stockport: Stockport Healthcare NHS Trust. Contact the front desk.
Tel: 0161 483 4398

Worthing and Southlands Hospitals NHS Trust (1997). *Good Practice Guidelines for Staff*.
Worthing: Worthing and Southlands Hospitals NHS Trust. Contact the press officer.
Tel: 01273 455622

Legal liability

Information producers may be liable in law for the consequences of the information they produce. If you are producing information for patients and members of the public, you need clear and detailed guidance about legal liability. The degree to which you or your organisation are liable depends on the aims of your information. For example, will your audience rely solely on your information to make their treatment decisions?

Methods you can use to protect against negligence claims include:

- using and quoting the source of good practice clinical guidelines
- making it clear what the information does and does not do, including disclaimers
- checking your organisation's insurance cover.

If you are thinking of using recognisable photographs or pictures of real people, make sure that they sign a disclaimer in which they agree not to have any ownership of your material. Model release forms can be obtained from the British Association of Picture Libraries and Agencies (*see* Useful contacts, p 103).

Case study: Examples of disclaimers

The following two examples of disclaimers provide an insight into some of the issues you need to consider. One is for a website and the other forms part of general information provided by an NHS trust. These anonymised examples are illustrative only, and should not be reproduced for your own organisation's use without appropriate legal input.

Example 1

Although every effort has been taken to ensure the accuracy of the information in this website at the time of publication, the organisation disclaims liability to any third party to injury damage or loss suffered as a result of reliance on the information in this website. Furthermore, whilst we have endeavoured to assess the quality of external sites that we have provided links to, we disclaim any responsibility for their content.

Links are provided for information and convenience only. We cannot accept responsibility for the sites linked to, or the information found there. A link does not imply an endorsement of a site; likewise, not linking to a particular site does not imply lack of endorsement.

While we have taken every care to compile accurate information and to keep it up-to-date, we cannot guarantee its correctness and completeness. The information provided on this site does not constitute business, medical or other professional advice, and is subject to change.

Example 2

Information supplied by the xxx NHS Trust. This information does not constitute health or medical advice and will not necessarily reflect current practice at xxx Hospital. If you have any questions about this information, please ask your doctor. No liability can be taken as a result of using this information.

Copyright

Copyright issues must be discussed and agreed before the information is produced. This is especially important if several different agencies are involved and where external funding has been obtained. Borrowing from published sources may involve issues of copyright – always contact the publishers of the material to be used for permission. Contact the British Copyright Council (*see* Useful contacts, p 103).

Informed consent

> @
> www.doh.gov.uk/consent

The NHS Plan promised a review of consent procedures to ensure that good practice in seeking consent for both treatment and research is in place throughout the NHS. 1 April 2002 was the date for the introduction of the new consent to treatment forms and accompanying patient information. The Department of Health's website makes available the full text of publications on consent being produced centrally. If you are writing a leaflet to support informed consent (for example, for a surgical procedure), it must meet the requirements of the Department of Health's *Good Practice in Consent Implementation Guide* and must include as a minimum:

- the aim of the procedure and intended benefits
- what the procedure will involve
- what kind of anaesthesia is likely to be used
- serious or frequently occurring risks if they exist for that procedure, and risks of doing nothing if applicable
- any additional procedures that are likely to be necessary (such as blood transfusion or removal of particular tissue)
- any alternative treatments that may be available if appropriate
- how long the patient will be in hospital
- what the patient will experience before, during and after the procedure, for example, details of the procedure, common side effects, pain relief if appropriate, and so on.

Confidentiality and use of patient data

Everyone who obtains information from particular patients and/or uses medical records of particular patients should be broadly aware of the general issues and policies that surround this topic. As producers of patient information can often come into contact with such information, the key papers and sources of further information are highlighted in this section.

> @
> The *Share with Care!* report is available at: www.nhsia.nhs.uk/ confidentiality/pages/ docs/swc.pdf

In 2002, the NHS Information Authority and Consumers' Association conducted some joint research to determine how people wanted their health information to be managed by the NHS. Confidentiality was the major issue reported, and just under a half of those questioned were reassured that their confidentiality would be protected by a published sharing agreement, which the NHS has agreed to deliver. Full details of this research and the wider issue can be found in the *Share with Care!* report (NHS Information Authority 2002).

@
HSG(96)18 and LASL(96)5 are available at: www.doh.gov.uk/ipu/ confiden/protect/ hsg9618.htm

In England, two health and local authority circulars, HSG(96)18 and LASSL(96)5, give guidance on:

- the circumstances in which information may be passed on
- keeping patients informed about the use made of information about them
- patients' right to access their own records
- information about children and young people
- security measures and retaining records
- dealing with patients who are offenders
- specific restrictions on passing on information.

@
www.doh.gov.uk/confiden/ cgmcont.htm

A further circular, HSC 1999/012, was issued in January 1999, following a key recommendation of the Caldicott Report (Department of Health 1999b). This report suggested that a network of organisational guardians should be established to oversee access to patient-identifiable information.

@
www.doh.gov.uk/ipu/ confiden/act/index.htm

In 2001, the Government passed the Health and Social Care Act. There has been much debate about Section 60 of this Act, as it gives the Secretary of State for Health the power to ensure that patient-identifiable data needed to support essential NHS activity can be used without the consent of patients. Further information about this (and the Patient Information Advisory Group, which was established to determine how the Act would apply in practice) is available at the Department of Health's website.

@
www.dataprotection.gov.uk

The Data Protection Act 1998 applies to personnel who are storing personal information in electronic or paper formats. The Act brings together the individual's right of access to information held about them, including their own health records. With the passing of the Freedom of Information Act on 30 November 2000, a new post (the 'information commissioner') was created to enforce the Freedom of Information and Data Protection Acts. An introduction to this, and guidance notes, are available on the information commissioner's website.

→ **Action points**

- Make sure that everyone involved in producing and providing patient information knows all the rules for using patient data and accepts responsibility for complying with them.
- Seek expert advice on the Data Protection and Freedom of Information Acts in advance if you want to set up any systems for collecting and storing information about named individuals.

Clinical Negligence Scheme for Trusts

The Clinical Negligence Scheme for Trusts (CNST), which is administered by the NHS Litigation Authority, reviews insurance cover for NHS establishments. Ten core standards are benchmarked and scored by a visiting assessor. Discounts on premiums can be given, subject to the score and level achieved.

Risk Management Standard 3 states that:

> *Appropriate information is provided to patients on the risks and benefits of the proposed treatment or investigation, and the alternatives available, before a signature on a Consent Form is sought.*

CNST General Manual (June 2002), p 35

To achieve the minimum level (Level One), CNST assesses whether such patient information is available for ten common elective treatments. To achieve Level Two, CNST assesses whether such patient information is available for an additional 20 procedures. The guidelines state that the information should answer certain questions depending upon whether it is information about a condition or a procedure.

Case study: 'CNST approved' information

A number of organisations, such as that illustrated here, produce information which has been 'CNST approved'. Use of such information may preclude the need to develop information in-house.

Eido Healthcare's INForm4U operation-specific, Informed Consent document library is a purposefully designed and developed risk management and patient information tool delivered on CD as PDF files.

The document library addresses all of the criteria stated in CNST's Risk Management Standard 3.

It has been written by specialist clinicians, with input from patients and patients' groups, and has been widely reviewed by both clinicians' and patients' representative organisations. It is in use in NHS Hospitals across the United Kingdom.

www.eidohealthcare.com

Source: Eido Healthcare website

Action points

- Find out whether your organisation has medical negligence cover and whether it covers your project.
- Consider whether the information you provide will comply with CNST's guidelines.

3 Planning an information package

Why do you want to produce information, who is it for and where can you find information that may already exist? These are some of the topics discussed in the first half of this section. The second half looks at project planning – timescales, teamwork, budgets and the like – and introduces the need for early thinking about dissemination.

Aims of your information package

It is important to be clear at the outset about the reasons for producing information for patients. The information itself should include a statement about its aims. You need to ask the following kinds of questions at the planning stage:

- Who is the package for (ie the target audience)?
- How can you ensure that it is relevant and useful to them?
- How do you think it will be used?
- What medium will be most attractive to the target audience?
- How will you ensure that the information can be easily understood?
- Does it fit the general aims of the organisation's information policy?

When you have discussed these questions with colleagues who will be helping you produce the material, write down your answers and turn them into a statement of aims. You may need to modify these preliminary aims as you go through the planning and piloting stages.

Defining the target audience

Think through exactly who you are aiming the information at. For example, many voluntary health organisations (such as the National Asthma Campaign) have been set up to provide support for people with certain illnesses or conditions and regularly produce information for their users. This kind of organisation knows its target audience, but still needs to consider whether one leaflet is suitable for all asthma sufferers or whether there should be separate materials for children, older people, different ethnic groups, or people affected by different levels of severity of asthma – mild, moderate or severe.

Another target audience could be patients in a group practice who want to know more about treatments for high blood pressure. Again, it is essential to consider the nature of the local population with high blood pressure. The topic you choose and its format should always match the wishes and needs of your target audience and your aims should be directed to their characteristics and needs.

Action points

Think through the aims of your information, considering the needs of the target audience.

- Take account of the organisation's information policy.
- Write down the aims, but be prepared to modify them in the light of preliminary discussions with patients and professionals (*see* Section 4).
- Clearly state your final aims in your information package.

Case study: Targeting your audience

The Terrence Higgins Trust produces a range of resources and takes great care to ensure that they clearly specify the target audience and the intended aims of each publication. In the following example it is clear who the material is for, why it is important to read it, and what it does and does not do.

---

2   **TERRENCE HIGGINS TRUST HEALTHY EATING GUIDANCE**

If you are HIV positive, healthy eating may not seem so important amongst all the other things you need to deal with. There is an old saying "You are what you eat" and a healthy diet can be a great benefit for everyone including you as a person living with HIV. This booklet will give you some practical tips on how to eat a healthy diet without trying to do a Delia and telling you how to cook.

Written by Andy Cooper

Based on original Nutrition research carried out by Nik Wendon – Daniels. Thanks to Gilead Sciences, Michael & Madeleine Daniels, David Watson and all those who financially supported the original research.

© Terrence Higgins Trust. May 2002 Charity reg. no. 288527

"Why is what I eat so important now that I have HIV?"

- A healthy diet is important for everyone, it doesn't matter if you have HIV or not.
- Combination therapy can have side effects, some of these can change how you feel about eating, and also you may have to eat certain foods before, after or with your drugs.
- Your body needs to be a strong as possible to fight infections and maintain health and well being.
- The best way of doing this is to make sure that what you eat is good for you, or at least not bad for you.

Source: Terrence Higgins Trust (2002)

Determining what information patients need

Organisations such as Patient Advice and Liaison Services (PALS), local NHS Direct call centres and local voluntary health organisations can help identify gaps in the current provision of health information. Medical audit and quality departments within NHS trusts and primary care trusts (PCTs) may be able to identify information needs through contact with patients and their carers.

Developing contacts

Contact a range of organisations to collect information on:

- local needs, whether they are currently being met and, if so, how and by whom
- local self-help groups and organisations representing people with particular health needs
- patient information that has been produced by other agencies relating to your area of concern.

Action points

- Listen to what patients, carers and health care professionals say about the kind of information they want – don't just rely on the questions they ask clinicians.
- Ask local audit departments what patients and health care professionals say about patient information.
- Ask local NHS trusts, PALS and PCTs what kinds of positive comments or complaints they receive from patients and carers relating to any aspect of information.
- Look at annual reports, local research and analyses of health information needs from the health authority.
- If you are in an NHS trust (in England), ask those who conduct the annual patient survey if they have any relevant information.

Further reading

Examples of recent UK studies on the information needs and information seeking behaviour of particular groups:

Biley A, Robbe I, Laugharne C (2001). 'Sources of health information for people with cancer'. *British Journal of Nursing*, vol 10, pp 102–6.

Couldridge L, Kendall S, March A (2001). 'A systematic overview – a decade of research. The information and counselling needs of people with epilepsy'. *Seizure*, vol 10, pp 605–14.

Davies MM, Bath PA (2001). 'The maternity information concerns of Somali women in the United Kingdom'. *Journal of Advanced Nursing*, vol 36, pp 237–45.

Drew A, Fawcett TN (2002). 'Responding to the information needs of patients with cancer'. *Professional Nurse*, vol 17, pp 443–6.

Echlin KN, Rees CE (2002). 'Information needs and information-seeking behaviors of men with prostate cancer and their partners: a review of the literature'. *Cancer Nursing*, vol 25, pp 35–41.

Jenkins V, Fallowfield L, Saul J (2001). 'Information needs of patients with cancer: results from a large study in UK cancer centres'. *British Journal of Cancer*, vol 84, pp 48–51.

Milewa T, Calnan M, Almond S, Hunter A (2000). 'Patient education literature and help seeking behaviour: perspectives from an evaluation in the United Kingdom'. *Social Science and Medicine*, vol 51, pp 463–75.

Mortimer CM, Steedman WM, McMillan IR, Martin DJ, Ravey J (2002). 'Patient information on phantom limb pain: a focus group study of patient experiences, perceptions and opinions'. *Health Education Research*, vol 17, pp 291–304.

Templeton HR, Coates VE (2001). 'Adaptation of an instrument to measure the informational needs of men with prostate cancer'. *Journal of Advanced Nursing*, vol 35, pp 357–64.

There have also been systematic reviews of the international evidence:

Forster A, Smith J, Young J, Knapp P, House A, Wright J (2001). 'Information provision for stroke patients and their caregivers'. *Cochrane Database Systematic Reviews*, vol 3, pCD001919.

Scott JT, Entwistle VA, Sowden AJ, Watt I (2001). 'Communicating with children and adolescents about their cancer'. *Cochrane Database Systematic Reviews*, vol 1, pCD002969.

The case study below exemplifies the many ways in which you can find out what information patients want.

Case study: Where does my information come from?

The *Guidebook for Ulcerative Colitis*, developed by Hope Hospital and Manchester University, has a fully referenced evidence base for each section, ranging from the general 'Introduction', through 'Taking enemas and suppositories', to 'Surgery'.

Evidence-based medical information was obtained through MedLine searches. Information on what patients wanted to know about ulcerative colitis was obtained from a number of sources (not included in the bibliography):

- directly from the patients themselves, through interviews and focus groups
- from searching the literature produced by patient support groups such as the National Association for Colitis and Crohn's and The British Digestive Foundation
- from the results of a phone survey conducted by the Medical Advisory Service in 1995
- from papers outlining surveys done to assess the demand for information (Martin *et al* 1992; Schlomerich *et al* 1987; Mayberry *et al* 1989; Din 1996; Ahmed 1997).
- from papers written by specialist gastrointestinal nurses outlining the information needs of their patients (Doughty 1994; Phillips 1995; Phillips and Warren 1985).

An insight into what patients want

Much of the research in this area indicates that patients want information that takes the following issues into account:

- **treatment options** – the information should include all treatment options, even if a scientific evidence base does not yet exist. This includes references to lifestyle changes (for example, diet) and alternative and complementary therapies
- **gaps and uncertainties about the scientific evidence** – where science doesn't yet have an answer, say so. Don't be scared to say 'We don't know'
- **quality of life** – this is of great importance to patients but not always fully considered by professionals. Patients want to know what it is like to live with a certain condition, not just the medical treatment options. They want to know how their condition or treatment may affect their ability to work, their usual activities, their family relationships and their sex life

- **inpatient services** – if a hospital stay is required, patients want to know about in-patient services, not just the operation itself. They want to know how to get to the hospital. Do they bring toothpaste? Can they have vegetarian food? Most hospitals now provide this kind of information for in-patients but you may want to include it as part of your package.

Further examples of other types of information, and useful prompts, are provided in Section 5.

→ Action points

- Make a list of all the aspects of treatment and care that will be of interest to your group of patients, taking account of the issues highlighted above.
- Use these points to identify the kinds of issues you will raise in your consultation with patients and carers (*see* Section 4).

Building on existing information

Seeing what others have done can save you work and give you ideas for improving what has already been developed, but remember that collating and reviewing existing information can also be time consuming.

- Ask organisations from the Useful contacts list (p 103) to send information relevant to your topic.
- Search some of the resources listed in Useful websites (p 117). If you don't have experience of searching online, most libraries will show you how to begin or may offer to do a search for you.
- Post a request to some of the online discussion fora listed overleaf, asking for any insights into information for your required area.
- If your patient group is likely to use social services or to need benefits, or your topic relates to social services, contact the local social services department to find out what information they produce.
- Ask patients and carers where they get their information and check what is offered in those places.
- Don't forget to ask your clinical or work colleagues, who may also be aware of unpublished material from their previous positions.

When you have collected a range of materials, assess each information package. Always check that:

- the clinical evidence base is accurate and up to date
- patients and/or carers have been involved in the design and content
- the material is relevant to your target audience and meets all their needs
- the information is readable and well presented.

If you identify any information that seems suitable, ask if it is available in languages familiar to the ethnic communities in your locality and in formats that are accessible for people with physical handicaps (especially those with sight and hearing impairment) and people with learning difficulties.

If you decide that existing material will meet your patients' needs, and that you won't have to develop your own, move on to Section 8 to consider how you will use and distribute it.

Action points

- Find out whether there is an existing information package that appears to meet your patients' needs.
- Use an assessment tool (such as Hi Quality – *see* p 86) to make sure that it is of good quality.
- Check that any information about clinical conditions and treatments is accurate and up to date.

Building on existing information, even within your own organisation, can be done and can reveal key hints on what to do and what not to do. The following example also suggests the need for an overall patient information policy to ensure quality and consistency across the trust.

Case study: Building on information

The Trust's Quality Assurance Steering Group agreed to adopt the audit recommendations and the first stage was a thorough review of all written patient information currently in use within the trust. This review was undertaken by the nursing development co-ordinator in order to identify gaps, compare leaflets and, importantly, to identify areas of good practice. In addition, details were obtained of when and where information was given to patients.

A very large collection of information leaflets was gathered with some clear outstanding examples of good quality production and content. Other leaflets available were poor quality photocopies of typed pages lacking details, guidance on how to seek further help and contact numbers. Basic information such as identification of the trust and department were also frequently missing.

Richardson and Moran (1995)

- Centre for Health Information Quality provides guidelines on reviewing health information
  @ www.hiquality.org.uk/guidelines.htm
- Lis-medical is an open discussion list for members of the UK medical/ health care library.
  Email: lis-medical@jiscmail.ac.uk
- Consumer Health Informatics is for those who are developing or evaluating electronic methods for the direct use of patients and the public. This includes patient education, information about services and other sources of help, and computer patient interviewing. Email: consumer-health-informatics@jiscmail.ac.uk
- Con-healthinc is a discussion forum for members of the Consumer Health Information Consortium (CHIC) and others with a professional interest in consumer/patient information. Email: con-healthinc@mailbase.ac.uk
- The NHS Plan requires each NHS trust in England to obtain feedback from patients about their experiences of care (see p 8). Some of these surveys may have identified information as an area for improvement and may provide insights into, and evidence of the need for, your resource development @ www.nhssurveys.org

Timescales

Decide when you want to complete the work. Base this on a realistic assessment of how long the process will take, bearing in mind the topic itself, the number of people available to help you and the amount of money you have to spend on the project. Experienced patient information officers say that it can take between three months and two years to create a finished product, depending on the complexity of the topic and the medium you have chosen.

Identify clear milestones within the overall timescale so that you can measure your progress throughout the project. For example:

- the date for the first draft to be finalised
- the date for the second draft to be discussed with patients and health care professionals
- the delivery date for produced materials
- the date for review.

Try not to underestimate how time consuming patient information production can be. If it is the first time you have produced information generally, or it is a new topic or medium, ask around to see what insights others can provide. The following example provides a loose benchmark:

> *The authors of this article have recently published an information pack on dysphasia, for patients and carers. Nursing home matrons, patients, carers and local health care professionals were canvassed to discover what information was required. The resulting booklet contains fewer than 1,900 words and took about 120 staff hours to write, spread over 14 months.*
>
> North, Magree *et al* (1996)

Teamwork

Think about whether you want to manage the project yourself – and whether you have the time and the relevant skills. Can one person manage the project or do you need to work with other people? It may be worth finding out if you have, or can get, the resources to support a full-time or part-time worker (*see* Paying for the work, p 28).

A number of agencies may be involved in the production of your patient information. Let them know well in advance what you plan to do and ask for their help – they can form part of your project team.

Think about what you may need, including:

- qualitative and/or quantitative research skills
- clinical expertise in your chosen topic
- an understanding of patients' information needs
- writing skills
- media expertise
- advice about evaluating your information.

Also consider the following questions:

- Are these skills available locally?
- Will you be able to afford to pay for them?
- Is there a local resource that could provide help without payment? (For example, art colleges sometimes want local design projects for their students – would your project be suitable?)

All the members of the project team, if you have one, must have clearly defined responsibilities and good channels of communication.

You may wish to consider setting up a steering group, or an editorial panel of experienced producers, to provide advice and guidance. The kinds of people you could invite to join the steering group include:

- academics with research experience
- members of the appropriate specialist voluntary health organisations
- representatives of the appropriate minority ethnic communities
- a PALS representative.

The following case study shows how a team in Nottingham that developed a children's bedwetting CD Rom came from a wide variety of professional backgrounds:

Case study: Working together

The multidisciplinary team that carried out the project involved academics and clinicians. A multimedia developer and a research assistant were both employed half-time for the 12 months of the project. The research assistant had a vital role in liaising between the two centres (academic and clinical).

To establish and maintain good teamwork and effective communication, monthly meetings were held at either the City Hospital or the Queen's Medical Centre throughout the project, to exchange information and express concerns (or congratulations) regarding the progress of the work. Minutes and agendas were circulated.

The nurse in charge of the clinic where the programme was being implemented was invited to all meetings, but was only able to attend a few. Involving the clinic staff in the development of the programme, as well its implementation, seems to have been appreciated and probably assisted with the acceptance of the computer in the clinic.

The console for the touchscreen was designed with clinic staff so they could move the computer equipment easily with minimal 'setting up' required, and there was little to be lost, damaged or stolen. It was decorated in an informal style so that children could recognise that the computer was there for them.

Remember that some of your consumer/lay members may require support and training in what may be new roles for them (*see* Further reading, p 38). It is useful to have support from senior management and clinicians (depending on your organisational structure). If you have received a grant from another agency, it will be important to keep them in touch with the work.

It can also be useful to link the project to policy initiatives, such as the NHS Plan or the Expert Patient initiative (*see* pp 8–9). These links can raise the profile of the project and may help if you need to apply for money.

Action points

- Get advice from previous information projects about their experiences. Contact the Centre for Health Information Quality, Consumer Health Information Consortium or the Patient Information Forum for advice from other developers of patient information. The more specific you can be with your request, the more results you'll see.
- Contact staff who have corporate responsibility for patient information (*see* Developing an information policy, p 12).
- Make sure that you have copies of all guidelines produced by your organisation that relate to any aspect of patient information.
- Link with current policy initiatives.
- Seek board and clinical support.
- Consider the need for an advisory group.
- Draft a realistic timetable, with milestones for each stage of the process.
- Identify the need for paid workers.
- Consider your budget and whether there is money to commission outside professionals for any parts of the work.
- Define the roles of all team members.

Looking ahead to dissemination

A common mistake people make at this stage is to put off thinking about how they will disseminate the material once it is produced. Planning a publicity and distribution strategy at the beginning of the work saves a lot of time and trouble at the end. It is also essential for budgeting: for example, you cannot budget for printing unless you know how many copies can be distributed and, therefore, how long your print-run needs to be.

Think about all the people who will be involved with the patient information package once it is produced and invite them to comment on your project and to suggest ideas for publicity now. As well as helping you think through your plans, the people you talk to will be more prepared to help at the end because they will probably feel more involved with the work and the final product (even if they never actually took up your initial invitation to contribute).

Publicity

Work out how much the publicity might cost and include a heading for it in your budget. Review all the different methods of publicising the material, including local radio, local newspapers, NHS journals, academic conferences, and the newsletters and other publications of national and local voluntary health organisations. Consider what you will be able to afford and which sources of publicity are free. For example, do you want to produce flyers to tell conference delegates about your information package, as illustrated below in the Nottingham bedwetting project?

Case study: The impact of publicity

The profile of the project has been raised in the public and academic domains through several channels. Thanks to the efforts of press officers of both the King's Fund and the University of Nottingham, there were several media reports about the developing project.

The national charity ERIC (Enuresis Resource and Information Centre) has been kept informed about the development of the project and even used the forthcoming education package to strengthen a bid for funds to the National Lottery.

Overall interest in the project is high. Approximately 80 leaflets about the project were picked up by delegates at the European Health Psychology Conference. Several clinicians involved in the care of children with nocturnal enuresis have made contact with members of the team to enquire about the availability of the package. Three paediatric consultants in the Nottingham area have approached the team with requests to put in for funding to develop and evaluate interactive multimedia patient information packages for the children in their care. Interest in funding for such a package is being shown by pharmaceutical and commercial publishing companies.

Distribution

Distribution can be costly, so think about the arrangements for delivering the materials to the distribution outlets. These may include local pharmacies, GP surgeries, libraries, NHS walk-in centres, outpatient clinics, wards, district nurses and community centres. For example, if you produce a leaflet, how will you supply people outside your local area? Are you going to charge a fee to organisations that request your information in this way?

 ## Action points

- Talk to people who are involved with public relations and communications locally or at the health authority.
- Draft a plan for publicity and distribution of the finished material.
- Take account of distribution when you are deciding how many copies of your materials to produce.
- Include the cost of publicity and distribution in your budget.

Paying for the work

It is easy to underestimate the amount of time and money it will take to develop a health information package. Some people may give their services free of charge; others will need to be paid. Even if your own organisation will pay for the production, distribution and publicity, it is worth working out a budget to make sure you have thought of everything. If you do this now, you should not be taken by surprise later on.

Costs might include:

- a paid project worker (and relevant training where necessary)
- fees for design, editing and illustrations
- translation
- collecting the views of patients and professionals (at various stages)
- piloting, external reviewing and media expertise
- production, including printing and reproduction
- publicity, dissemination, distribution
- support
- evaluation.

People sometimes forget to budget for hidden costs and overheads, such as stationery, photocopying, writing applications for money, advertising for posts, servicing the steering group, databases searches and buying in other expertise, such as information technology. For example, involving patients and professionals using any of the methods mentioned in the next section – such as focus groups – is essential, but can be costly.

Case study: The need for accurate estimates

A Redbridge and Waltham Forest Health Authority project on anxiety aimed to promote the mental health of Asian women in Redbridge. To do this, the team planned to adapt and translate two existing English booklets – one on depression, the other on anxiety – into four Asian languages.

However, when initial estimates for the cost of translation were compared with real quotes, it was realised that insufficient funds were available to allow both booklets to be developed. This resulted in the project team re-appraising their overall project aims and deciding to deliver only one adapted and translated resource – on anxiety.

Finding money to support your project will vary according to where you work. It is important to identify where the funding came from to make it clear that the cost of production has not been met at the expense of core services and that it has not come from sources that have not been 'approved' by NHS trusts or health authorities. Some NHS organisations have policies that exclude accepting money from pharmaceutical companies (*see* Sponsorship, overleaf).

Case study: Sample costings

In October 2001, a leading London-based voluntary health organisation produced an A6 sized, seven-page (14-sided), full-colour concertina booklet.

The costs for 30,000 copies of the publication (of which 20,000 were distributed free by another organisation) were as follows:

Project staff/management	£6,325
Illustration	£500
Design	£1,100
Print	£3,600
Distribution	£400
Corporate overheads	£3,625
User involvement	£730
Total	£16,280

Please note that staff and overheads may be lower in a more volunteer-based organisation, or those with offices outside London. However, distribution might cost more in another field as this voluntary organisation already has a major national publication provided free of charge to many people with the condition, and it distributes through its already established regional networks.

Within NHS trusts, you could approach your manager for information about endowment funds and whether your project could be eligible to apply for any. Funding may be available through local policy initiatives such as public health or patient partnership.

Sources for project funding (p 114) lists some funding bodies and reference sources. Contact possible agencies before you start to write the application. Writing a proposal for financial support takes time and you should make sure that you know what each funding agency requires from an application. Many funding bodies now encourage open dialogue to assist potential applicants in their submissions, and produce written guidance about their funding priorities and application procedures.

Colleagues who have already made applications for research grants or sponsorship may be willing to share information about the agencies they have approached and offer advice about writing applications.

Sponsorship

Your project may be eligible for sponsorship from a pharmaceutical, or other commercial, company. English health authorities have recently redrawn their guidelines about dealing with this industry and you should check what your organisation's policy is before you decide to approach, or accept sponsorship from, any pharmaceutical company. It is also advisable to gain consent from the chief executive (or equivalent) before pursuing arrangements with commercial organisations.

---

i

The Health Coalition Initiative (HCI) works to develop relationships between pharmaceutical companies and voluntary health groups. It may be a useful source of advice and contacts if you are unfamiliar with either of these organisational groups (*see* Useful contacts, p 103).

Further reading

Health Action International (1999). *The Ties That Bind: Weighing the risks and benefits of pharmaceutical industry sponsorship* @ www.haiweb.org/campaign/spon/toc.html

Long-Term Medical Conditions Alliance (1998). *Working with the Pharmaceutical Industry.* Guidelines for patient organisations considering whether to approach pharmaceutical companies for financial help. Covers working with the industry and acknowledging its support. Updated in June 2000 @ www.lmca.demon.co.uk/docs/pharmgds.htm

→ Action points

- Make a list of all the things you will need to do to develop your material.
- Estimate how much it will cost. If necessary, get help from a financial manager or someone else in your organisation who has experience of doing similar work.
- Consider and approach external sources for funding (*see* Sources for project funding, p 114).
- Check guidelines before agreeing to a sponsorship deal with a commercial company.

Support and training

It is always worth looking round for other people, in your own organisation and in local NHS trusts or voluntary organisations, who may have relevant experience. Nurses and people who work in quality departments can be helpful as they often have experience of putting information together. Some trusts now have patient information officers you can contact for advice.

On a national level you should contact the Patient Information Forum, Consumer Health Information Consortium or the Centre for Health Information Quality (*see* Useful contacts, p 103). Sharing experience with other producers usually gives you lots of tips and ideas and can help solve some of the problems you may be having. Help is only a phone call (or email) away. If you would like to learn more about producing patient information, a selection of organisations that run training courses is provided in the Information point, below.

ⓘ

- **The Centre for Health information Quality (CHIQ)** runs health information appraisal training to raise awareness of quality issues for providers and producers of health information in order that the quality of the end product is enhanced. The two key workshops offered are 'Producing good quality information' and 'Patient Advice and Liaison Services (PALS)'. Further information **@** www.chiq.org/chiq/training_new.htm
- **The Patient Information Forum (PiF)** has information about training courses on patient information developed by members for personnel within their own NHS trust.
- **The Plain English Campaign** also runs a wide range of courses on writing in plain English and a specific course on making medical jargon more simple.
- **The BMA Library** runs several courses focusing on finding and appraising evidence, and using the internet. Further information **@** www.bma.org.uk/ap.nsf/Content/_Hub+library+training+courses
- **The British Library** produces a web page providing a good single source about information courses, including the CILIP courses plus others in the field, including those involving consumer health information **@** www.bl.uk/services/information/training.html
- **The Critical Appraisal Skills Programme** aims to help you find, appraise and act on evidence, through workshops, open learning, e-learning and other support. It is also looking at further developing patient information workshops that use DISCERN and CHIQ's Hi Quality Guidelines (see p 85).

Support

Think how you will support the package once it has been distributed. How will you ensure that the information you produce is correctly displayed, or that it is distributed at the correct time to the correct patients? Will you need to designate a contact point for people who want to ask questions after they have received the information? Suppose people find it difficult to load your CD Rom on to their computer? How will you make sure that people who have received the information also receive updated versions as you produce them?

 Action points

- Arrange internal and external support services, such as distribution.
- Consider the implications that information will have on patients and professionals.
- Plan your technical support.

Implications and consequences

The final thing to consider in your planning is the knock-on effect that informing patients may have on services. Will patients expect a choice of treatments where only one was offered previously? It is worth discussing these possibilities with senior members of your organisation and, where appropriate, the local health authority.

Case study: Knowledge is not necessarily power

Informed Choice leaflets were specially produced to provide women with up-to-date, high quality information on choices they could make during their use of maternity services. However, the results quoted directly from the research paper show that despite excellence in leaflet production, organisational and professional barriers prevented full utilisation of this resource.

- *Health care professionals were positive about the leaflets and their potential to assist women in making informed choices, but competing demands within the clinical environment undermined their effective use.*
- *Time pressures limited discussion, and choice was often not available in practice.*
- *A widespread belief that technological intervention would be viewed positively in the event of litigation reinforced notions of 'right' and 'wrong' choices rather than 'informed' choices.*
- *Hierarchical power structures resulted in obstetricians defining the norms of clinical practice and hence which choices were possible.*
- *Women's trust in health care professionals ensured their compliance with professionally defined choices, and only rarely were they observed asking questions or making alternative requests.*
- *Midwives rarely discussed the contents of the leaflets or distinguished them from other literature related to pregnancy.*
- *The visibility and potential of the leaflets as evidence based decision aids was thus greatly reduced.*

Stapleton *et al* (2002)

4 Collecting the evidence

This section explains the importance of involving patients and professionals in developing your information and outlines some of the ways in which this can be done. It then outlines the importance of ensuring your clinical information is up to date and suggests a range of sources to ensure this is so.

Patient and carer views

These days, when people talk about 'evidence' in a health care context, they are usually referring to medical evidence. Increasingly, however, there is acceptance of the position long held by social scientists that the views and experiences of patients and carers may inform what they want to know about their illnesses, conditions and treatment. If collected rigorously, these views are another essential aspect of evidence.

In order to meet this broader definition of evidence, organisations that develop guidance are now extending their literature searching coverage. For example, the Scottish Intercollegiate Guidelines Network (SIGN), when reviewing a clinical topic, in addition to medical evidence now also looks for studies that include patients' and carers' views on:

- positive and negative experiences of the condition, including diagnosis, medication and other treatments
- unfulfilled needs
- information needs, preferences and choices
- participation in decision making about treatment choices and preferences
- overall satisfaction with care received.

@
www.show.nhs.uk/sign/
patients/index.html

Genuine involvement or consultation with patients, users and carers will result in a far more useful information package – after all, they are the ones who will be using it. It is rare that consumer goods (such as a car or washing machine) would reach the market without some form of consumer testing. Why should patient information be any different?

Involving patients throughout the process will help you to produce information that best meets their needs. For example, health care professionals can tell you what the signs and symptoms are of a chronic condition, but it's only patients themselves who can tell you what it's actually like to live with it. Given that perspective, you'll understand why even a well-presented and evidence-based publication may still fail to answer the questions patients are asking.

Involving users from the start of the project is essential and an important criterion for the quality of the resources, and indeed of the process itself. There are five main stages where patient and carer input is essential:

Stage one
The preliminary stage for checking your ideas (*see* Section 3).

Stage two

Once you have decided to go ahead and produce your own information package, you should collect the views of patients and carers about:

- where they have received previous information and what they thought about it
- the content of information they would ideally like to have
- where and when they would like to have it
- what format they would like it to be presented in (for example, in writing, as a leaflet, or visually as a video – *see* Section 6).

Stage three

When you have prepared the first draft of your information package, discuss what patients and carers think about the material or test it out with them in a process sometimes called piloting (*see* Running a pilot scheme, p 90).

Stage four

Once the content of your material is finalised, again seek their views during the review period.

Stage five

After the information has been in use for some time (for example, after one or two years), it will need evaluating, and possibly updating (*see* Section 9).

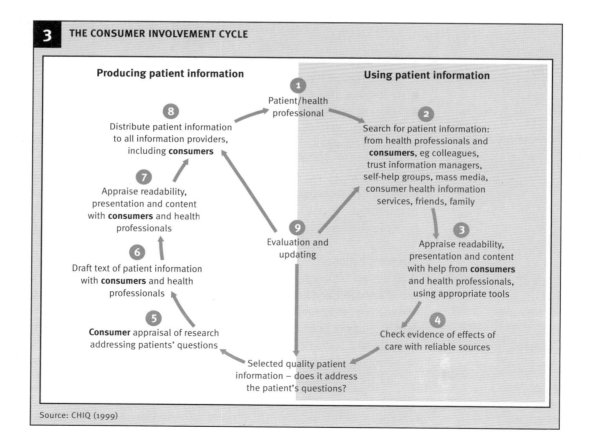

3 **THE CONSUMER INVOLVEMENT CYCLE**

Producing patient information

Using patient information

1 Patient/health professional

8 Distribute patient information to all information providers, including **consumers**

2 Search for patient information: from health professionals and **consumers**, eg colleagues, trust information managers, self-help groups, mass media, consumer health information services, friends, family

7 Appraise readability, presentation and content with **consumers** and health professionals

9 Evaluation and updating

3 Appraise readability, presentation and content with help from **consumers** and health professionals, using appropriate tools

6 Draft text of patient information with **consumers** and health professionals

5 **Consumer** appraisal of research addressing patients' questions

Selected quality patient information – does it address the patient's questions?

4 Check evidence of effects of care with reliable sources

Source: CHIQ (1999)

Planning your involvement

Before you select a method for consulting with patients and carers, think about the following factors:

- What kinds of people do you need to involve (for example, newly diagnosed patients or existing patients, their families and carers)? Select a group of patients that is sufficiently wide to encapsulate the appropriate range of views. Patients chosen through a voluntary organisation may not be typical of 'ordinary' users. Indeed, the very fact that they have joined already shows an increased awareness and interest in the area.
- What range of people do you need to involve, for example older people, younger people, people with disabilities, men or women or both, minority ethnic groups? (*see* Section 6).
- Will you need to use sampling methods? If so, which tools are most appropriate, for example a questionnaire, a topic guide or a series of open-ended questions?
- What form of analysis will you use once you have collected the views of patients? Will you need help with the analysis? Will you use existing computer software for the analysis, and if so, which is the most appropriate software, and is it easily available to you?

And now for a few tips:

- If you do not have experience of research and sampling methods and analyses, ask for advice. Local academic or audit departments may be helpful.
- Listen carefully and honestly to what people say – don't just look for confirmation of your ideas.
- Give feedback to the people you involve. As well as a basic courtesy, it is important for them to know what the findings are. It could affect their lives.
- Keep the patients informed of progress and provide them with copies of the draft and final packages.

Lastly, before you make any final decisions, check with your Local Research Ethics Committee (if you don't where they are, try COREC – *see* Useful contacts, p 103) to see if you need their approval for this kind of research. In some cases you may do, and this involves writing and submitting an application to the committee. Find out what their timetables are. Sometimes this process can take a long time – as much as six months – and can hold up the development process.

Collecting views of patients and carers

There is a wide variety of ways in which to collect people's views and the list below is not comprehensive, but it will provide you with an outline of the main methods and sufficient detail to conduct one, or a range, of them. Don't let unfamiliarity prevent you from involving patients in your development – seek help from experienced colleagues if you need to.

Focus groups

Focus groups involve selecting up to 12 people from the groups who will be using the information. They are useful because:

- they enable you to collect the views of patients and carers quickly
- they provide an open-ended forum where people can exchange and share their views

- they are a particularly effective method of brainstorming and generating ideas about improvements
- they gather a range of views over a short time, and the breadth of experience of the people involved provides a sound basis on which to build further work.

The discussions need careful planning and a topic guide. This is a prepared list of the topics and questions you need to explore to find out what patients and their carers want from the information material. A sample topic guide can be found in the appendix of *Informing Patients* (Coulter *et al* 1998).

A skilled facilitator is essential for running the group. Discussions should last for one to two hours. Make sure the proceedings are recorded. Someone trained in focus group analysis should analyse the transcription. Offer participants expenses and ideally give them feedback on the results of the exercise.

Despite your good intentions, some patients may not wish to participate in focus groups. For example, in one project some children (and in some cases, their parents) were too embarrassed to join in discussions about the development of a multimedia system on the topic of bedwetting. In such a situation, you would be better to use one of the other methods outlined below.

Case study: Using focus groups to improve *The Cancer Guide*

For this study BMRB Qualitative used focus groups, an established qualitative technique (also known as group discussions), to explore the views of cancer patients for Macmillan Cancer Relief. Five such groups took place around Britain. A series of in-depth telephone interviews (ten in all) were also conducted to make sure that people unable to attend the focus group had an opportunity to participate in the research.

Each focus group involved nine or ten people and lasted just over two hours. Respondents were keen to take part in the research, and people who were unable to take part were often disappointed that they could not participate.

Each focus group was audiotaped and transcribed verbatim for subsequent analysis.

All the respondents (with the exception of one who was a carer) were people who had direct experience of cancer at some point in their lives, usually within the previous three years.

Mindful that people from different cultures or backgrounds have different needs with regard to information and how it is delivered, one focus group was held with people from minority ethnic groups.

Further reading

Centre for Health Information Quality (1999). *Involving Consumers in the Development and Evaluation of Health Information*. Winchester: Centre for Health Information Quality. Provides an example (based on lower back pain) of the process of developing good quality, evidence-based information that meets the needs of the patient.

Coulter A, Entwistle V, Gilbert D (1998). *Informing Patients*. London: King's Fund. Provides examples of how focus groups were used with 62 patients to assess the quality of 54 existing patient resources (leaflets, videos, and audiotapes).

Entwistle VA, Watt IS, Davis H, Dickson R, Pickard D, Rosser J (1998). 'Developing information materials to present the findings of technology assessments to consumers. The experience of the NHS Centre for Reviews and Dissemination'. *International Journal of Technology Assessment in Health Care*, vol 14, pp 47–70. p63 highlights some of the issues of working with different voluntary health organisations, and how they may have their own agenda to promote.

Surveys

Surveys are used to gather information about patients' views, usually through a questionnaire. They have the advantage of allowing information to be collected from large numbers of people and, if properly designed to reach a random sample of patients, offer statistical reliability and validity.

Write the questionnaire carefully so that the questions do not bias the responses, and so that they are easily understood by the people for whom they are intended. If you have little or no experience of writing questionnaires, ask for help with the preparation. If a previously validated questionnaire matches your needs, use that instead, or use it as a basis upon which to develop your own.

Once you have drafted it, the questionnaire should be piloted with people who have the same characteristics as the target group to be used in the main sample.

Surveys can be administered using interviewers who ask the questions on a one-to-one basis, or by sending the questionnaire to named individuals by post. The analysis of the data that is collected is usually done using a computer software package. These packages allow relatively fast descriptive results and statistics.

In-depth interviews

Interviews with individual patients or carers provide a wealth of information about what people want and need from health care information. They are usually carried out by trained interviewers using a checklist of topics, allowing people to give spontaneous replies in their own words, which are recorded on tape. People often feel more comfortable in this situation, but interviews are time consuming, and the analysis of respondents' data is often more complex than with focus groups.

Other methods

Other methods of collecting information include:

- **the Delphi technique** – involves gathering a number of individuals together (virtually in some cases) to pool their collected wisdom about specific topics
- **panels** – regular meetings of a selected group of patients to give their views about health care locally and how it can be improved for users
- **observation of specified processes** – for example, outpatient clinics, or consultations between patients and their doctors.

Each of these methods has advantages and disadvantages, but the important thing is to select one or more methods that are most appropriate for your topic and situation. If you have little or no experience of research, ask for advice. University departments and independent research agencies will often be prepared to help. The Further reading section below provides additional insights into this area.

→ Action points

- Decide which groups of patients, users and carers you need to involve and consult.
- Choose the most appropriate methods to collect patient and carer views.
- Check with your Local Research Ethics Committee to find out if you need their approval.
- Collect and analyse data.
- Give feedback on the results to patients/carers and to the professionals involved.
- Use the results to inform the first draft of the material.

Further reading on patient and public involvement

The Welsh Health Circular (WHC (2001) 83). *Signposts: A practical guide to public and patient involvement* contains details on how the above should be done, and operational guidance and project management tips on how to undertake patient and public involvement. It includes sections on the advantages and disadvantages of different techniques, signposts to references and sources of support and chapters on building capacity to do the work (for example, supporting patients, changing organisational culture and joint working) @ www.wales.gov.uk/signposts

Barker J, Bullen M, DeVille J (1999). *Reference Manual for Public Involvement*. London: Bromley Health Authority. Provides guidance on a broad range of issues (from Bromley Health).

Health Education Authority (1999). *Positive Participation: A planning and training resource*. London: Health Education Authority. Encouraging more effective involvement of young people in health promotion activities.

Kelson M (1997). *User Involvement: A guide to developing effective user involvement strategies in the NHS*. London: College of Health.

Kohner N, Leftwich A (1998). *Partnerships: A training pack*. London: Health Development Partnerships. An imaginative, stimulating training pack on skills for partnership with patients and clients with lots of good practical workshop exercises.

National Consumer Council/Service First Unit (1999). *Asking Your Users: How to improve services through consulting your consumers*. London: National Consumer Council. A guide to consulting public service users, including a summary of methods of consultation.

National Consumer Council (2002). *Involving Consumers in Healthcare*. London: National Consumer Council @ www.ncc.org.uk/pubs/pdf/case_study_health.pdf
Identifies challenges such as:
- adopting a strategic approach to consumer involvement
- sharing good practice
- taking practical steps to involve disadvantaged and marginalised groups
- clarifying the role of 'lay' members.

The Tizard Learning Disability Review, Vol 2 (1997) (Brighton: Pavilion Publishing) and the NHS Executive's good practice guide *Once a Day* (March 1999) @ www.doh.gov.uk/nhsexec/onceaday.htm provide examples of consulting with people with learning difficulties.

---

i

The *User Involvement Research* mailing list aims to bring together people with expertise in user involvement and public participation in the evaluation and delivery of public services. Email: user-involvement@jiscmail.ac.uk

---

Collecting views of professionals

Although this guide deals with information for patients, it is important to incorporate and assess the views of professionals. In this context, the term 'professional' includes not only clinicians but also managers and receptionists, for example, all of whom will provide useful views on processes such as inpatient procedures.

In many situations, it is the clinicians who are in a position to identify and disseminate your resources to patients and to discuss it with them. Expert knowledge is essential in many cases where up-to-date evidence about clinical conditions needs to be incorporated into the information.

It is necessary to implement similar stages of involvement to those already described for patient and carer involvement. Professional views should be collected at all stages of production – planning, collecting views, and testing out material.

Entwistle *et al*'s case study reproduced below demonstrates the importance of obtaining professional feedback on the accuracy of the factual content of your information (*see* Clinical evidence, overleaf), and on its presentation and appropriateness of use.

Case study

Professional views

All leaflets were informed by the best available research evidence about the effectiveness of the interventions and by some evidence about the context into which they would be introduced and the information needs of the intended audience.

All leaflets were peer reviewed both by people able to comment on the congruence of the information presented with the best available research evidence and by those able to comment on the likely suitability and usefulness of the information material to their intended users.

Entwistle *et al* (1998)

Action point

- Collect the relevant professional and clinical views on the material at all stages of production (in other words: planning, involvement, testing and review) in the same way that you have collected the views of patients and carers.

Clinical evidence

As mentioned in Section 3, one of the key elements that patients wish to see in patient information that covers conditions (such as asthma and diabetes), and associated tests and investigations, is what options exist for treatment and/or intervention. Many patients want to understand how much is known and what is not known and the relative risks and benefits of each of the treatment options. These options can include lifestyle changes, complementary and alternative therapies and doing nothing (also known as 'watchful waiting'). In order to provide these answers, look for the latest evidence in the topic you are covering.

> @
> http://minerva.minervation.com/cebm (go to Levels of evidence)

Evidence means that your information has to be based upon well-conducted systematic reviews or well-conducted primary research if reviews are unavailable. To assess the validity of different types of primary research, there are guides to the hierarchy of evidence (for example, the JAMA user guides and the Centre for Evidence Based Medicine website).

> @
> Evidence-based guidelines are also available at:
> www.sign.ac.uk
> www.guideline.gov/index.asp
> www.nelh.nhs.uk/guidelinesfinder

It is as important for patients to be aware of this evidence as it is for clinicians. One of the first problems that people experience is how to find the most up-to-date research. The sources of help provided in the Information point opposite should get you started, but the task can be daunting if you don't have experience of this kind of work. You may find it helpful to talk to clinical specialists in your locality. Ask them, for example, if you could have a copy of any evidence-based clinical guidelines that they use and if they would be prepared to explain anything in them that you don't understand.

Because clinicians themselves often find it difficult to keep up to date, you may need go to some of the sources listed below to find answers to the particular questions that have arisen, and to make sure that what you have is accurate.

One of the next considerations is to ensure that the evidence you collect is applicable to the audience you have identified. There is little point in collecting evidence on the treatment of asthma in adults if your audience is made up of children under 12. In addition to age, think about things like gender, ethnic background and disability.

Who to contact

> @
> Additional resources are available at:
> www1.york.ac.uk/inst/crd/em51_app1.htm
> www1.york.ac.uk/inst/crd/em51_app2.htm
> http://minerva.minervation.com/cebm

Searching for the best quality clinical evidence is a specialised task and, unless you have those skills, you will need help. Places where you can find this kind of help locally include:

- public health departments, medical schools and some university departments (statistics and psychology, for example)
- audit/quality departments within NHS trusts
- librarians.

See also Training, *opposite.*

Further reading

Booth A (1997). *The ScHARR Guide to Evidence-based Practice*. Sheffield: University of Sheffield.

Booth A (1998). 'Information about health technology assessment'. *Evidence-based Health Policy and Management*, vol 2, pp 30–1.

Booth-Clibborn N, Milne R, Oliver S (2001). 'Searching for high-quality evidence to prepare patient information'. *Health Information Libraries Journal*, vol 18, pp 75–82.

The following is a list of some of the specific organisations and projects where you may be able to find the evidence you need:

- **The Cochrane Library** is the best place to start. It contains the **Cochrane Database of Systematic Reviews** which provides abstracts of reviews and titles of reviews in progress. The database can be searched for specific words and phrases or browsed by Collaborative Review Group @ www.cochrane.org/cochrane/revabstr/mainindex.htm or, for NHS professionals @ www.nelh.nhs.uk/cochrane.asp
  Free access is available through the National electronic Library for Health @ www.nelh.nhs.uk/cochrane.asp
  The database is one of several in the Cochrane Library listing research findings. There is a specific site for the Consumer Collaboration Consumer Network @ www.cochraneconsumer.com
- **The TRIP database** @ www.tripdatabase.com attempts to bring together all the 'evidence-based' health care resources available on the internet. At the latest count, in February 2002, there were approximately 29,000 links from nearly 70 sources. The site is updated monthly.
- **Bandolier** is a monthly news-sheet and website giving up-to-date information about clinical evidence @ www.jr2.ox.ac.uk/Bandolier
- **The NHS Centre for Reviews and Dissemination (CRD)**, at York University, offers a free online database search service to help UK enquirers identify systematic reviews and economic evaluations. It also offers free databases of systematic reviews, economic evaluations and health technology assessments @ www.york.ac.uk/inst/crd/welcome.htm
- **Clinical Evidence**, from BMJ Publishing, is a compendium of the best available research findings on common and important clinical questions, updated and expanded every six months @ www.evidence.org or free @ www.nelh.nhs.uk for NHS professionals. It is also freely available to everyone in England through the National electronic Library for Health @ www.nelh.nhs.uk/clinical_evidence.asp, which also produces the bi-monthly *Effective Healthcare Bulletins.*
- **The National electronic Library for Health** provides information to NHS staff on clinical guidelines, National Service Frameworks and the TRIP database @ www.nelh.nhs.uk
- **The Directory of Clinical Databases** @ www.DoCDat.org is a free information resource that enables enquirers to find out rapidly whether a database suitable for their needs exists. Users can search on a wide number of criteria, ranging from the type of patient, condition or treatment to the geographical area covered.
- **UpToDate** @ www.utdol.com is a US subscription-based clinical information resource that is updated quarterly and claims to provide concise, practical answers for physicians when they need them the most – at the point of care. It is reputed to be similar in nature to Clinical Evidence and recent trials at Portsmouth Hospitals, which allowed NHS-wide access to it via the web, received a number of favourable reports/requests for continued access.

Health promotion

The Health Development Agency (HDA) specialises in producing systematic reviews of public health evidence, including reviews on current knowledge of what works in tackling health inequalities, in areas such as obesity, smoking, mental health, mobility in later life and HIV @ www.hda-online.org.uk/evidence

Complementary and alternative therapies

The Research Council on Complementary Medicine (RCCM) provides information on the evidence base for complementary medicine based on rigorous research to encourage safe and effective practice and improved patient care (*see* Useful contacts, p 103).

Training

- The Critical Appraisal Skills Programme (CASP), along with the Finding the evidence Programme (CASPFew), have produced two evidence-based health care open learning resources to help users find and make sense of evidence: an interactive CD Rom with workbook and a paper-based resource of five separate units. Further details from CASP. *Also see* the support and training Information Point, p 31 (*see* Useful contacts, p 103).
- A new publication entitled *Literature Searching: A user guide* has been produced by Library and Information Services at the Chartered Society of Physiotherapy. The full publication is available as a free download @ www.csp.org.uk/libraryandinformation/publications/view.cfm?id=258

Clinical guidelines

Guidelines aim to improve the quality of health care for patients by reducing variation in practice and outcome. They consist of statements that assist practitioner and patient decisions about what health care is appropriate for specific clinical circumstances.

There are many guidelines available, but most are based on a consensus of 'expert opinion' or a non-systematic review of the scientific literature. Evidence-based guidelines are derived from a systematic review of the scientific evidence, and are therefore less susceptible to bias in their conclusions and recommendations.

- **Scottish Intercollegiate Guidelines Network (SIGN)** seeks to involve consumers, and their evidence, in the development of all their clinical guidelines @ www.sign.ac.uk
- **The Australian National Health and Medical Research Council (NHMRC)** has produced a handbook, *How to Present the Evidence for Consumers: Preparation of consumer publications* (2000) which focuses on how to prepare guideline information in a way that consumers can readily access and understand. It is based on a 1999 review of the relevant scientific literature about how to prepare and present evidence-based information for consumers of health services @ www.health.gov.au/nhmrc/publications/synopses
- **Prodigy** is a broad concept to support general practice in developing the quality of clinical practice. It includes reference material on approximately 131 conditions @ www.prodigy.nhs.uk

Entwistle V, Watt IS, Herring J (1996). *Information about Health Care Effectiveness*. London: King's Fund.

Glanville J, Haines M, Auston I (1998). 'Finding information on clinical effectiveness'. *BMJ*, vol 317, pp 200–3.

Greenhalgh T, Donald D (2000). *Evidence-based Health Care Workbook: For individual and group learning*. London: BMJ books.

Guyatt G, Rennie D eds (2002). *Users' Guide to the Medical Literature: A manual for evidence-based clinical practice*. Chicago: American Medical Association.

Holmes-Rovner M, Llewellyn-Thomas H, Entwistle V, Coulter A, O'Connor A, Rovner DR (2001). 'Patient choice modules for summaries of clinical effectiveness: a proposal'. *BMJ*, vol 322, pp 664–7.

Kubba H (2000). 'An evidence-based patient information leaflet about otitis media with effusion'. *Clinical Performance and Quality Health Care*, vol 8, pp 93–9.

Conflicts of interest

It is important to find out whether local practices vary from national standards or guidelines in case individual patients are not told about the full range of options available, or are not advised that local practice conflicts with national practice.

Also think about some of the possible conflicts of views between professionals. There have been examples of good quality patient information being developed where some professional health care professionals disagreed with some of the evidence base and the way this information was presented. In a project about childbirth, for example, a leaflet was produced that contained evidence about statistics for ultrasound in early pregnancy. The ultrasonographers strongly disagreed with the way in which these statistics were presented (Oliver *et al* 1996). See the case study on p 32 for further insights into this project.

There may also be differences of views between what patients have told you and what professionals think. In such situations you should inform each party of the views of the other, and attempt to reach a compromise. If this doesn't work, the final decision will have to be made by you or an independent arbiter.

Alternatively, the information you produce should make it clear where there are uncertainties, ambiguities and differences between professional views and patient views. If something is not known, say so! This will allow patient and professionals to openly discuss the issues and (hopefully) come to a mutual agreement.

→ Action points

- Discuss ways of finding good quality clinical evidence for your topic with two or more of the following:
    - librarians and specialist information services
    - clinical colleagues
    - public health specialists
    - academics
    - audit departments
    - clinical governance leads.

@

www.bma.org.uk/ap.nsf/
Content/__Hub+library+
training+courses

- Libraries are key sources of help in searching for clinical evidence – the BMA Library runs several courses focusing on finding and appraising evidence and on using the internet.
- Talk to local clinicians and people who have skills in making technical language easy for people to read and understand.
- Check local practice and practice guidelines for variations from national standards.
- Ensure the material explains all treatment options, even if local practice does not include some of them. Patients are entitled to know that other options exist – including non-intervention (in other words, doing nothing).
- Carefully consider how to inform patients of non-evidence-based approaches such as complementary therapies.
- Make it clear where uncertainties and ambiguities exist – if you need to, say 'we don't yet know'.

Presenting the evidence

When you have collected the clinical evidence, spend some time thinking and talking about the best ways to present it for patients. The language used in the sources of evidence is often technical and not easily understood by lay people – it will therefore need to be rewritten. You should also consider the kinds of references you wish to provide for patients who want to follow up your information package with some further reading.

Some of the things you should take into account are:

- the order in which the information is presented
- the way in which the messages are put over – positive, negative, or mixed (*see* Section 5)
- the way in which statistics and probabilities are explained
- the best way to present graphical information
- the way in which all the treatment options are described (including complementary and alternative therapies (*see* the Case study below) and the option of non-intervention)
- how the gaps and uncertainties in the evidence are presented.

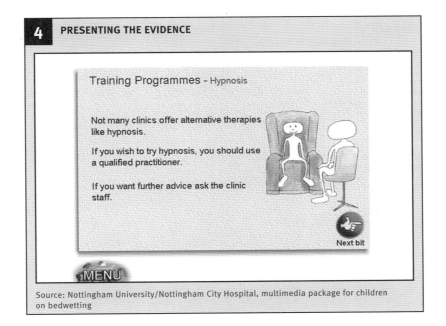

Source: Nottingham University/Nottingham City Hospital, multimedia package for children on bedwetting

Further reading

Edwards A, Elwyn G, Mulley A (2002). 'Explaining risks: turning numerical data into meaningful pictures'. *BMJ*, vol 324, pp 827–30.

Entwistle VA, Watt IS, Davis H, Dickson R, Pickard D, Rosser J (1998). 'Developing information materials to present the findings of technology assessments to consumers. The experience of the NHS Centre for Reviews and Dissemination'. *International Journal of Technology Assessment in Health Care*, vol 14, pp 47–70.

5 Content and presentation

This section presents a number of generic items that need to be considered when producing resources, depending on the setting in which they are used. Once you have outlined these, you will need to consider how to tie them together, so this section looks at writing style and readability. Lastly, it considers some key points regarding the presentation of material and look at the Department of Health's new guidelines for the presentation of patient information as part of its NHS Identity work.

Using the information and activities suggested in Sections 3 and 4, you'll now be able to list most, if not all, of the aspects of treatment and care that are of interest to your audience. In the following pages we list some examples. However, they are unlikely to cover the variety of topics and types of information package you are producing and should be treated as prompts. Some are only relevant to certain settings or particular types of information.

Key information

Unless you have a good reason for excluding them, all the following items should be considered when preparing your information:

Clinical information

- simple description of condition
- prognosis and clinical outcomes
- brief overview of treatment options, including non-intervention
- benefits of the proposed treatment or investigation (impact on quality of life)
- risks, possible complications and side-effects of treatment (impact on quality of life)
- clear and unambiguous statements about preparation for specific procedures
- why the treatment is needed and how to prepare for it
- what happens during the treatment and how long it takes
- expected levels of pain and discomfort and advice about dealing with them
- sensory information – description of the range of possible sensations that patients are likely to feel
- description of the care required following the procedures
- dos and don'ts on going home, including advice about rest, time off work, everyday activity, sexual activity, pain relief, alcohol, bowels or using the toilet, driving, lifting, bathing, sickness certification
- length of recovery phase and how patients may feel at each stage to full recovery if this is achievable
- when and where to seek further professional advice.

Inpatients

- name of consultant and named nurse (where possible, use generic posts so the leaflets can still be used when staff change)
- where to go and who to ask for more information or to answer questions
- ward routines, including visiting times, facilities and whether companions and children are welcome
- what to bring and what not to bring
- likely length of stay
- what happens after discharge
- department address, telephone, email, fax, minicom numbers
- if the patient is worried, who they should contact for more information or to answer questions
- clear directions to the department, including parking and a detailed map of the department and site.

Outpatients and day cases

- full names of consultants and specialist clinics (where possible, use generic posts so the leaflets can still be used when staff change)
- directions, transport details and whether people can travel home alone, whether they are likely to be fit to return directly to work, child care, and so on
- how much time to allow, and what will happen
- details of planned investigations, tests and how results are given
- whether students are likely to be present
- names and contact details for changing appointments or to get more information.

Additional information

Where applicable, also consider providing details of:

- how to give positive feedback or make a complaint
- details of the local PALS
- NHS Direct or NHS 24 service (0845 4647 in England and Wales, 08454 242424 in Scotland)
- details of local self-help groups
- their stage in NHS journey, in other words a map of where they are in the health system (*see* p 69 for an example)
- relevant health promotion material and sources for further reading
- who is providing this information material, where and when (this should include author details and their qualifications)
- who was involved in the development process, for example 'This leaflet was tested with 35 patients and reviewed by two specialists in [discipline].'
- reference sources for factual statements
- month and year of publication
- list of key points, contents page, glossary
- a tear-off slip for comments (*see* p 97 for an example, or the final page of this guide).

In addition to information on conditions and services, patients and users are increasingly requesting further information in a range of specific areas, such as:

- medicines
- clinical trials
- performance tables
- copying referral and discharge letters to patients.

Information on medicines

If you are preparing information on medicines, ask the legal department of the Royal Pharmaceutical Society for advice. From a policy and patient involvement perspective you should also review the work of the Medicines Partnership Task Force, which is taking forward the concept of concordance – a new approach to the prescribing and taking of medicines based on partnership between patients and professionals.

The **Electronic Medicines Compendium** is an excellent source of UK medicines information. It lists the patient information leaflets (PILs or package inserts) that pharmaceutical companies produce to accompany their products and provides online access to useful resources such as the **British National Formulary (BNF)**, which is updated twice a year.

@
http://emc.vhn.net

Remember where possible to use generic names (for example, paracetamol) as opposed to proprietary names for medicines, as this will reduce the number of changes necessary when new products are released or brand names are changed.

A number of groups specialise in the production and provision of medicines information. For example:

@
www.aiopi.org.uk

@
www.medicinechestonline.
co.uk
www.hsis.org (Health
Supplement Information
Service)
www.chic.org.uk (Consumer
Health Information Centre)

@
www.abpi.org.uk

@
www.ukmi.nhs.uk

- **The Association of Information Officers in the Pharmaceutical Industry (AIOPI)** is the professional organisation for individuals in the industry who are involved in the provision and management of information.
- **pecmi** looks to improve information for consumers around the supply of medicines in the UK, both prescription and self-medication.
- **The Proprietary Association of Great Britain (PAGB)** produces a range of resources focusing on over-the-counter medicines and food supplements.
- **The Association of the British Pharmaceutical Industry (ABPI)** provides a range of publications. The 'Target' series covers a range of conditions and has been developed in partnership with voluntary health organisations, many of which are listed on the Links page of its website.
- **UK Medicines Information** is an information resource and portal to other medicine information repositories intended primarily for health care professionals in primary and secondary care.

@
See a recent example at:
www.informED.org.uk

UK pharmaceutical companies are bound by legislation that currently restricts the amount of medicines information they are able to provide to consumers. Some companies provide general health information through educational grants to relevant voluntary health organisations (*see* Sponsorship, p 30).

Many voluntary health groups and other organisations produce medicines-related information. For example:

@
www.aidsmap.com

@
www.rcpsych.ac.uk/info

@
Available at:
www.which.net/health/dtb/
treatment.html

- **NAM Publications** produces a range of factsheets on anti-HIV medication
- **The Royal College of Psychiatrists** produces an excellent factsheet on antidepressants and on a range of conditions, some of which are also available in Chinese
- **The Consumers Association** has also produced patient-friendly versions of their professional-focused *Drug and Therapeutics Bulletin*. These are called 'Treatment Notes' and were developed after the Consumers Association spent months not only working out how best to present scientific information in patients' terms, but also how language, font size and style, colour, pictures and other layout issues can be used to enhance readability. There is a charge for these publications.

Further reading

Barber N (2001). 'Ensuring patients' satisfaction with information about their medicines'. *Quality in Health Care*, vol 10, pp 130–1.

Haynes RB, McDonald H, Garg AX, Montague P (2003). 'Interventions for helping patients to follow prescriptions for medications' (Cochrane Review). The Cochrane Library, Issue 1.

Information on clinical trials

This is an area in which the quality of information, or lack of it, is coming under increasing scrutiny. The following case study exemplifies some of the issues, and solutions in this area.

Case study: Improving patient information for clinical trials

The pharmaceutical company Novartis produces information sheets for patients taking part in clinical trials of new medicines. Novartis commissioned Consumation, a consultancy specialising in health information design, to ensure their information sheets and consent forms were as user-friendly as possible and review their current practice.

Consumation started by following the Research Ethics Committee template, as the committee reviews all information sheets. It then suggested some initial changes to the formatting, layout, sequence and vocabulary. Finally it tested the draft for readability, comprehensibility and effectiveness using the European Commission's guideline for testing patient information leaflets, entitled *A guideline on the readability of the label and package leaflet of medicinal products for human use* (29 September 1998).

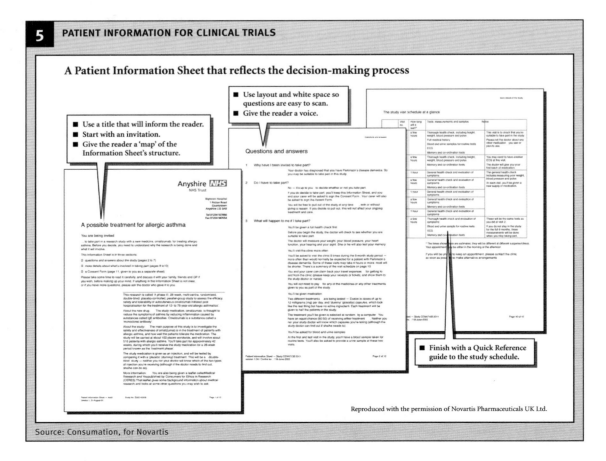

Source: Consumation, for Novartis

The new Novartis model has the following special features:

- It follows the sequence of the patient's own decision-making process.
- It groups related items of information together.
- It offers readers a clear, hierarchical structure with clear signposts for navigation.
- It provides a clear, concise overview on the front page.
- Its structure allows patients to choose a level of detail matching their particular needs and preferences.
- It summarises the timetable of clinic visits in a single-page 'at-a-glance' guide.

The work has resulted in model text that improves patient understanding of complex concepts and – to judge by users' comments – appears to ease the anxieties of potential participants.

---

i

A quality tool for this sort of information is being developed at Leicester University (*see* TriLET, p 86)

Further reading

CancerBACUP (2002). *Understanding Cancer Research Trials (Clinical Trials)*. London: CancerBACUP. Booklet addressing the many questions people ask about cancer clinical trials.

CERES (1994). *Spreading the Word on Research. On writing patient information leaflets*. London: CERES. This is a practical booklet for researchers, ethics committee members and others who write or assess information for people asked to take part in research
@ www.ceres.org.uk/publications.htm

Hanley B, Truesdale A, King A, Elbourne D, Chalmers I (2001). 'Involving consumers in designing, conducting, and interpreting randomised controlled trials: questionnaire survey'. *BMJ*, vol 322, pp 519–23. Study that found that input from consumers helped improve the quality of patient information.

@
As part of this 'patient choice' work, more information is being provided on the range of local services available, star ratings and waiting times, primarily at: www.nhs.uk

Other non-NHS organisations also provide 'performance' or location type information, including: www.drfoster.co.uk

http://healthmap.co.uk/

www.specialistinfo.com

Presenting performance tables

The NHS Plan clearly states that patients will be given access to information that allows them more readily to measure the performance of their doctor and other NHS services.

@
www.doh.gov.uk/ patientprospectus.

Each PCT was required to deliver a booklet entitled *Your Guide to Local Health Services* (also known as the Patient Prospectus) to every household in their geographical boundary during October 2002.

Copying letters to patients

In England, both the Kennedy Report and the NHS Plan (*see* p 8) mention the need for referral and discharge letters to be copied to patients. The NHS Plan, Section 10.3 states: 'letters between clinicians about an individual patient's care will be copied to the patient as of right' (Department of Health 2002a, p 89).

The two key issues to consider are content and presentation. Clinicians need to phrase technical medical jargon in terms that patients can comprehend. Those responsible for

See the *Toolkit for Producing Patient Information* at: www.doh.gov.uk/nhsidentity

presentation (patient information officers, communications staff, receptionists and the like) must pay attention to corporate guidelines, such as those recently issued under the NHS Identity banner.

Further reading

Chantler C, Johnson J (2002). 'Patients should receive copies of letters and summaries'. *BMJ*, vol 325, p388.

Full details of above Department of Health initiative can be found through the Patient Letters Working Group @ www.doh.gov.uk/patientletters

The NHS Learning Zone provides advice on writing letters for patients @ www.doh.gov.uk/learningzone/letters.htm

→ Action points for content and presentation

- Clearly state who your information is for, the scope and the aim of the information package (as outlined in Developing an information policy, p 12).
- Make a list of all the points you think should be included in the 'ideal' information package.
- Check out ideas informally with other colleagues and some patients/carers to get a better idea of the important items you should include and how much support there is for your plan.
- Weigh up the amount of support there is from health care professionals and patients. No one information package can meet everybody's needs.
- Depending upon this, and on the findings of your user involvement exercise, list the topics on clinical issues and/or services your information will cover.
- Patients like case studies and stories of other patients. You can gather these from your own or colleagues' experience or from the patients themselves. Remember that you must never name names or include details that will enable people to identify either patients or health care professionals.

These are also available from the Database of Individual Patient Experience at: www.dipex.org.uk

Telling the story

After listening to patients and collecting the clinical evidence (*see* Section 4), bring together all the topics you have decided to include. For more comprehensive information packages (such as booklets or CD Roms), plan how you will communicate this information by designing a storyboard. This involves arranging the information into a 'story' that will make sense to lay people, with a beginning, a middle and an end.

You can order your topics in many different ways. For instance:

- Start with what is most important to the patient.
- Tell the story in the order that the patient will experience it.
- Take different themes in turn (such as causes of the illness or treatments).
- Address the topic from the point of view of different patient characteristics (for example, young people or older people).

At the end of each section, think about what you want your patients to be able to do. You can use a summary to emphasise the most important issues and help patients to remember key points.

→ Action points

- Collate the evidence (both patient-related and clinical).
- Before you begin writing your first draft, put yourself in the shoes of one of your patients. Try to answer the following questions from that patient's point of view:
  - What am I experiencing physically right now?
  - How long have I been experiencing this?
  - What practical effect has this had on my life in terms of my work, finances and social activities?
  - What effect has it had on me and my relationships with my partner, family and friends?
  - What is my emotional state right now?
- Construct a storyboard.
- Set deadlines.
- Circulate for comment.

Case study: A multimedia storyboard

The Misbehaving Bladder project at the Bristol Urological Unit in Southmead Hospital developed a useful storyboard technique for keeping track of all the various resources required to develop their multimedia package on urinary urge incontinence. The diagram below, produced for the project by MEdIT Ltd, illustrates how this was incorporated into their Development Process.

The storyboard was specifically designed for the development of a multimedia package. However some of its key stages, such as script, patient feedback, peer review and evaluation, are core to most resources.

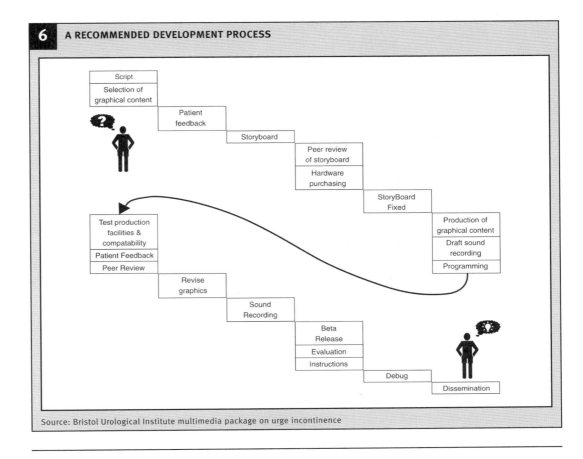

6 | A RECOMMENDED DEVELOPMENT PROCESS

Source: Bristol Urological Institute multimedia package on urge incontinence

Choosing your writing style

Your style creates an impression that underlies everything you say, and it gives away a lot about how you regard patients. It is really important to make people feel comfortable from the start. Show that you recognise the patient as a whole person who has feelings as well as a medical condition. A few words at the beginning of your introduction will do. If you have difficulty, imagine that you are talking to a friend or sending them a letter.

Keep the following key principles in mind:

- **Use positive images** of minority ethnic groups, older people, women, people with physical and learning difficulties, people with mental illnesses and other groups who may face discrimination and prejudice. You can get advice and examples of positive images from specialist organisations looking after the interests of these groups:
  - Commission for Racial Equality for ethnic groups
  - Council for Disabled Children
  - Equal Opportunities Commission for women
  - Age Concern or Help the Aged for older people
  - MIND for people with mental illnesses
  - Royal National Institute of the Blind (RNIB)
  - Royal National Institute for Deaf People (RNID).

> *i*
>
> Local branches of these organisations are usually listed in the telephone directory and the national offices are listed in Useful contacts, p 103.

- **Use words and images that won't exclude people** because of literacy levels, gender, socio-economic backgrounds, age, physical or mental ability, race, culture or sexual orientation. Avoid masculine and feminine words.
- **Don't make assumptions**. Avoid words and images that assume that all families have two parents. Don't assume everyone is heterosexual and married – the term 'partner' is more inclusive than husband or wife.
- **Avoid defining groups of people by their illness**. Do not refer to people as manic-depressives, diabetics or epileptics. Instead, refer to 'people with manic depression', 'people with diabetes' or 'people with epilepsy'.
- **Remember the special needs** of people with visual and hearing impairments. Also remember that people with these difficulties also have medical conditions that are not related to their impairments (*see* Section 6).
- **Most statements should be in the affirmative**. 'Give only when the patient wheezes' is clearer than 'Do not give unless the patient is wheezing'. Use negative sentences only to emphasise when an action should be avoided.
- **Information about treatment effects can highlight the positive or the negative aspects**. An 85 per cent chance of survival is also a 15 per cent risk of dying, and a treatment that relieves symptoms in 90 per cent of cases does not relieve symptoms in 10 per cent of cases. Think carefully about whether you want to highlight the positive or the negative message, or present both (*see* Further reading, p 59, for more on risk communication).
- **Instructions should be specific rather than general**. 'Take one tablet three times a day 20 minutes before meals' rather than 'Take three times a day'.
- **Use familiar words, not jargon**. If you need to use medical terms, explain them when they are first used and provide a glossary of terms.
- **Do not abbreviate or use acronyms**. Using initials or abbreviations may confuse and irritate your audience. If it is unavoidable, explain what they stand for when you first use them, as follows: primary care trust (PCT).

◼ Case study: Starting with empathy

Coming into hospital can seem overwhelming at first, but we would like you to feel welcome and we will do everything we can to make you feel comfortable. We hope that this leaflet will answer some of your questions and help you settle more easily into the ward. And if there is anything else at all that you would like to know, please do ask us!

Al Brookes, former Patient Information Project Worker, Brighton Health Care NHS Trust, 1997

Plain English

- Use short words, short sentences and short paragraphs. Short words are more likely to be included in the vocabulary of people with low literacy skills. Short sentences, listing the main points using numbers or bullet points, make the information easier to understand. They also increase the chance that people will read on. Short paragraphs, expressing a single idea, with sub-headings for each section, enable the reader to concentrate on one message or point at a time.
- Use the active voice rather than the passive. For example, 'take the medication', rather than 'the medication should be taken'.
- Be direct. 'Do not take this medicine with any other drugs' tells the reader that it is their own responsibility to avoid other drugs. 'This medicine should not be taken with any other drugs' sounds more like a suggestion or advice.
- Take a personal approach. Say 'the nurse or doctor will ask you to lie down' (using the second person), rather than 'the patient will be asked to lie down' (using the third person).

Readability

Consider whether to use published readability factors (RFs), such as The Gunning Fog Index, Gobbledygook, Watchword and the Flesch test. Some word-processing programmes (Microsoft Word, for example) have readability scores built into their software. However as the Raynor Backwards test shows, they may be of limited value and the readability score alone does not indicate the appeal and impact of a leaflet (*see* the FPA Case study below).

Raynor Backwards Test

An inappropriate emphasis is given to RF. They are based on word and sentence length (or word difficulty) and take no account of layout, typeface, motivation of the reader, or previous knowledge. It is salutary to note that any passage would receive the same reading score whether it was written forwards or backwards.

Raynor (1998)

◼ Case study: Scores are not everything

In the FOG readability test, a Family Planning Association (FPA) leaflet scored well on readability with 10, yet the non-FPA leaflet had a lower score of 9.2. (Examples of scores are: news story in tabloid paper 10, broadsheet newspaper 17, an insurance policy 20.) Yet the FPA leaflet was much preferred. It is apparent that a straight readability test does not give the whole picture, as it does not reveal interest, relevance or humour which make young people more inclined to start and continue reading.

A word of caution

Please remember that no matter how many guidelines one follows, not everyone can write well for patients. It may be better to approach someone within your organisation who you know has the appropriate skills in this area, or to find someone external who may able to assist.

If you choose someone to write the information for you, make sure they are fully briefed on what they are to write, and for whom. Ask to see examples of work that have previously done which matches your brief as closely as possible. Also make sure that any costs are agreed in advance, including subsequent modifications to their original manuscript.

See also Quality standards (p 82) and Section 6.

The following organisations may be able to help you find a writer:

- Association of British Science Writers: www.absw.org.uk
- Guild of Health Writers: www.healthwriters.com
- Media Medics: www.media-medics. co.uk
- Medical Journalists Association: www.medicaljournalists. org.uk
- Society of Authors: www.writers.org.uk/ society
- Society of Medical Writers: www.lepress.demon.co. uk/home.htm

Resources from Designers in Health's April 2002 study day on information design, plus a useful reading list, are available to download @ www.dihnet.org.uk/events

Presentation

Issues such as page size, typeface and type size, line length, justification and use of colour can be so detailed that it is not possible to deal with them fully in this guide. However, the Department of Health guidance on writing, printing and producing patient information is reproduced opposite. It is important to note that it is always worth consulting a professional graphic designer about presentation and layout so that you produce the most effective information package within your budget.

Some printers work with graphic designers and you could also consider approaching NHS Supplies, the medical illustrations department, or local arts and technical colleges, if appropriate. Alternatively, contact the Institute of Medical Illustrators (which has instituted a new award (*see* p 94) or ask Designers in Health, whose email discussion list comprises about 150 designers and communications professionals working in health care.

Case study: The effects that fonts can have on readers

The phrase 'You are invited to Fiona's party' was laid out in Flash B Bold font and again in Palatino Italic font. One participant got Palatino Italic, the other got Flash B Bold. Each was asked to read out what the card said to confirm to the group that the words were identical. Each was then asked in turn what they would wear to the party. The one who had Flash B Bold said informal, while the one with Palatino Italic said formal. The only difference was the typeface. A simple test, but very effective.

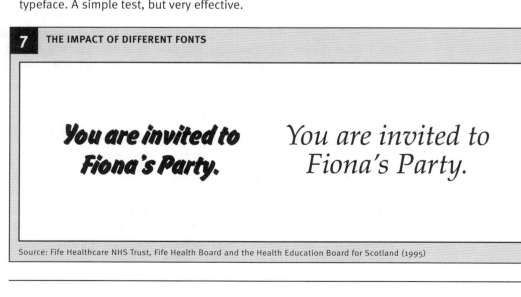

7   THE IMPACT OF DIFFERENT FONTS

You are invited to Fiona's Party.

You are invited to Fiona's Party.

Source: Fife Healthcare NHS Trust, Fife Health Board and the Health Education Board for Scotland (1995)

Depending upon your organisational structure, colleagues in other departments, such as Communications, Marketing or Quality, may be able to, or indeed need to, assist in specifying corporate presentation standards (*see* Developing an information policy, p 12). The Department of Health has developed written guidance and supportive templates to make it easier for the NHS to produce good quality information that meets the needs of the patient and the public, as well as its own requirements. It is called the *Toolkit for producing patient information.*

---

i

The Toolkit is available online @ www.doh.gov.uk/nhsidentity.
For a hard copy, contact the NHS Responseline. Tel: 0870 155 5455 quoting ref 29682.

The following extracts are from Section One:

Extracts from the *Toolkit for Producing Patient Information*

4 General guidance on writing patient information

To make text more inviting to read, use the following:

- **Short sentences** – *in general no more than 15 to 20 words long.*
- **Lower case letters**, *where possible, as they are easier to read. Exceptions to this are proper names and the first letter in a sentence.*
- **Present and active tenses**, *where possible, for example, 'your appointment is on...' not 'your appointment has been made for...'*
- **A question and answer format** *is helpful to divide up text.*
- **Bulleted or numbered points** *to divide up complex information.*
- **Small blocks of text.** *Do not use long paragraphs, divide them up using headings and new paragraphs.*
- **White space** *makes the information easier to read.*
- **Large bold font** *emphasises text. Avoid UPPER CASE letters, italics and underlining as they make the text more difficult to read.*
- **Numbers** *from one to nine are more easy to read if they are written as words, and numbers from 10 can be represented as numbers.*
- **A font size** *of no less than 12 pt (see the print guidelines).*
- **Diagrams and pictures** *are very effective and should be in line with our communications principles. Where appropriate, use them to illustrate the text, remember to label them and do not print over them. You should not use clipart as it does not add to the reputation of a professional organisation.*

6 Presenting written information for patients – printing and production check list

The more clear, inviting and good quality a leaflet looks, the more likely it is that people will read it. All our information must be clearly identified as coming from us with our logo on the front cover. This will make it easier for the patient to recognise what is and isn't part of the NHS.

We have produced templates for you to use, or for you to give your printer to use, these are in Section 2.

Leaflet style and format

- *Folded leaflet – size $\frac{1}{3}$A4 (DL), six or eight pages (approximately 800 or 1200 words but less if diagrams are included).*
- *Longer leaflets should be produced in A5 size.*
- *Leave space between the paragraphs and do not have too much text on the page.*

- *Make sure that headings are clear.*
- *The weight of paper should be 130 to 150 grammes per square metre (gsm).*
- *Ideally, the paper should be matt to prevent light reflecting off it.*

Consistent features

Front cover
Anytown Healthcare NHS Trust and logo
Title of leaflet, for example, Gastroscopy
Department or directorate where appropriate, for example, endoscopy unit, womens'
health

Back cover
Website address
Date of publication
Leaflet code
Copyright note of organisation.

Print guidelines
You should apply these principles to all documents, not just those for people with sight difficulties. A large number of patients using the NHS will be over 40, and clear, legible print with the lines not too close together will make documents easier to read.

- *Font size: 12 point (minimum) to 14 point, but if you are writing information for the elderly or people with sight difficulties always use 14 point or larger.*
- *Use a medium weight typeface, for example Frutiger Roman or Medium.*
- *Contrast: use a light background with dark print.*
- *It is acceptable to use a dark background with white print (reversed out) for headings, but not for a large body of text.*
- *Use a sans serif font – Frutiger.*
- *Justify the text to the left only.*
- *Use one or two colours.*
- *Do not write text over background pictures or a design.*

NHS (2002)

→ Action points

- Decide where to go for design expertise, and commission the work.
- Check the design and layout with patients and colleagues.
- To find a quality printer, ask colleagues in your own and other local organisations. Get at least two estimates from different printers and ask to see recent examples of their work. Look for quality, not just price. Consider using your local medical illustrations department.
- Decide on the number of copies. Think about how large your audience is, how you will be able to distribute copies, and when you will next need to update the material. Consider whether it is preferable to produce a large number of cheap copies to a smaller number of a higher quality.
- Ask for advice on the best production method, including:
  - **size and format:** an A5 booklet or one-third A4 pamphlet is convenient for patients to carry around and refer to
  - **print production process:** for 500 or fewer copies, it may be cheaper to use 'docutech' (a digital printing process straight from a computer disk) where the price per copy is the same however short or long your print-run. For longer print-runs, you can make considerable savings by litho printing (a traditional printing process from film) because the more copies you print, the lower the price per copy

- **photocopying**: if you have to rely on photocopying, ensure that it is always done from a master copy of consistent quality, laminated (if necessary), and used only for leaflets that are produced in small numbers (up to 300 copies)
- **the colour and type of paper** to be used for inside pages and for the cover (weight, shiny or matt, recycled or newsprint)
- **binding and additional requirements**: for example, a pocket for enclosures (having a pocket adds about 30 per cent to the cost)
- **colour of ink** (using two colours adds about 10 per cent to the cost of using just one)
- **source and style of illustrations** (for example, photos, line drawings, charts or diagrams)
- **design**: avoid flashy fonts, graphics and colours
- **source and style of illustrative material, tables and extracts**.

---

8 | **BRIEFING A DESIGNER; FOUR WAYS OF TREATING THE SAME DESIGN**

Briefing a designer

The designer, assuming you decide to use one, will visit you to discuss your needs. They will want to know:
- who will be reading the booklet – in this case, patients and their relatives or friends
- what size and how long you want the booklet to be
- whether you want it to be printed in one colour or more (black counts as a colour)
- whether you want illustrations
- whether your hospital has any logostyle, symbol or 'house' colours such as the castle in the Castleport booklet
- the dates when you want the booklet to be completed and delivered.

Four ways of treating the same piece of graphic design, all in one colour

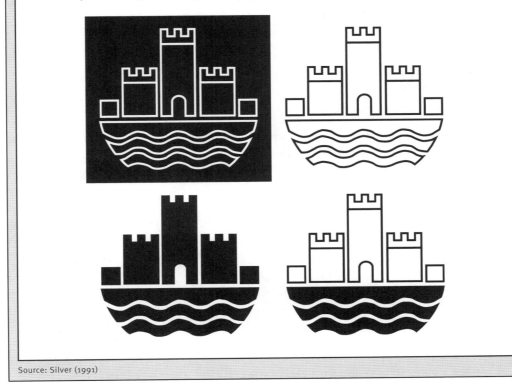

Source: Silver (1991)

Further reading

Entwistle V, O'Donnell M (1999). *The Guide to Producing Health Information*. Aberdeen: Aberdeen University. Online guide to producing health information including an excellent section on information needs and gaps in research evidence
@ www.abdn.ac.uk/hsru/guide.hti

Getting Your Message Across is a pack produced in 1995 by (the then) Fife Healthcare NHS Trust, Fife Health Board and the Health Education Board for Scotland. It started from the point of view that non-designers (and in this case non-Health Promotion Officers) were going to write and produce patient information. A small number of packs, priced at £49.95, are still available.

Salford Centre for Health Promotion (1994). *Getting it Right When You Write*. The Salford guidelines for written information about health.

Secker J, Pollard R (1995). *Writing Leaflets for Patients: Guidelines for producing written information*. Edinburgh: Health Education Board for Scotland. Free of charge to health promotion and health education specialists.

Plain English

Training and guides on clear health care writing are available from a range of providers, including *The Plain English Guide to Writing Medical Information* from the Plain English Campaign, or Tim Albert Training (*see* Useful contacts p 103).

Beenstock J (1998). *In the Clear*. South Manchester University Hospitals Trust's account of providing jargon-free information written in plain English, with a simple questionnaire to ensure patients' views are taken into account.

Foundation of Nursing Studies (2001) *Plain Words for Nurses: Writing and communicating Effectively*. London: Foundation of Nursing Studies. This is an educational tool to advise on effective writing and presenting techniques and is specifically written for nurses, midwives and health visitors and other health care professionals.

Wilson R (1998). *Ensuring the Readability and Understandability and Efficacy of Patient Information Leaflets: PILS project summary report*. Newport: Sowerby Centre for Health Informatics at Newcastle (SCHIN).

Readability

Centre for Health Information Quality (1998). *The Advantages and Disadvantages of Readability Tools*.

Ewles L, Simnett I (1995). *Gobbledygook. Promoting health: A practical guide*. London: Scutari Press.

Flesch RE (1948). 'A new readability yardstick'. *Journal of Applied Psychology*, vol 32, pp 221–33.

Meade CD, Smith CF (1991). 'Readability formulas: cautions and criteria'. *Patient Education and Counseling*, vol 17, pp 153–8.

Petterson T (1994). How readable are the hospital information leaflets available to elderly patients? *Age and Ageing*, vol 23, pp 14–6.

Presentation

Wright P (1999). 'Designing healthcare advice for the public', in *Handbook of Applied Cognition*, Durso F ed, pp 695–724. Chichester: John Wiley & Sons.

Risk

Calman KC (2002). 'Communication of risk: choice, consent and trust'. *Lancet*, vol 360, pp 166–8.

Garrud PWM, Stainsby L (2001). 'Impact of risk information in a patient education leaflet'. *Patient Education and Counseling*, vol 40, pp 304–7.

6 Choosing the medium

This section looks at what medium best suits your audience. It identifies issues that you need to consider when collecting their views earlier in the process and discusses specialist audiences (such as those with learning difficulties) before reviewing the different types of media that exist.

i

Some of the information in this section is reproduced from *Getting it Right When You Write*, with kind permission from the Salford Centre for Health Promotion.

Your choice of medium will be influenced by:

- who the audience is, their preferences and needs
- the nature of the information and the message to be communicated
- access to technical expertise
- funding and resources.

As new media are developed, the same basic criteria need to be applied in assessing whether they are the most appropriate and effective way to communicate specific information to a specific audience. Does the use of information technology sufficiently enhance the delivery of the message to justify its use over paper?

Who is your audience?

Your information should truly represent and reflect the needs of its intended audience.
To choose the most appropriate and effective medium, find out about:

- **your target audience** – their age, gender, linguistic, educational and cultural background, sensory or other impairments
- **the number of people you expect to reach** – for example, the cost of producing multimedia materials means that they are not likely to be appropriate unless the information is to reach large numbers of patients
- **how the audience will want to use the resource** – will they use it once only, or repeatedly as a reference source? Will they want to pass it on to family/ friends?
- **where the material will be used** – by patients on their own at home, or by groups of patients in a clinic or hospital with the support of a facilitator who can respond to questions and concerns
- **the context in which the material will be used** – material designed for people going into hospital has a different context from that designed to stop people from smoking, or for coping with illness.

Responding to patients' preferences

Include the choice of medium in the discussions during your user involvement exercise (*see* Section 4). Ask patients to say how they would like the information to be presented and balance this with the resources you have. If possible, give them a choice of formats – do they want to see a video, read a book, or hear a tape? Be honest about what you can provide and be willing to change your own ideas about what you think may be best for them.

Think about using more than one medium. When considering resource implications, think about the ways that information prepared for one client group (for example, large print for people who are visually impaired) may also be useful for others (such as people with learning disabilities or people whose first language is not English).

Patients like the opportunity to make a contribution while they use the information package. It is often assumed that only multimedia packages can be interactive. However, paper-based packages can also offer opportunities for patients to add in their own observations. Leaving sections for the patient to fill in with details – such as their own name, their GP's contact details, appointment dates, their questions, and a record of their own progress – helps them to feel that they are more involved with the management of their own condition.

The figure below shows an example of some patient-held record sheets used in the *Guidebook for Ulcerative Colitis* developed at Hope Hospital and the University of Manchester.

Source: Manchester University/Hope Hospital, multimedia package on colorectal cancer

Targeting minority groups

People whose first language is not English

Written information may not be suitable for ethnic communities who cannot read written English. Depending on the age and gender of the target group, some of them may not necessarily read or write in their own first spoken language. Translation is not an add-on. Whether you are producing a leaflet, an audio cassette or a video, it must be considered from the beginning of the project, and taken into account when you decide which medium to use for your information and when you draw up your budget.

Translation is not about taking information produced in English and simply converting it into another language. In some languages, literal translations for English concepts do not exist and translators cannot provide a word-for-word substitution. Sometimes the explanation provided by the translator may distort the meaning, and discrepancies should be discussed fully so that the translator can give an accurate description of a concept for which there is no exact translation.

Case study: 'You don't speak my culture'

Many Asian women in Redbridge were unfamiliar with the term 'depression' to describe their clinical condition. They considered that they were suffering from a thought sickness – *soochnee ke bimaari* – a sorrow in the heart. Faith and spiritual healing is a common treatment option for this condition in their own culture but is not considered by western cultures.

Redbridge and Waltham Forest Health Authority anxiety project

It is necessary to consider cultural differences between western and other models of medicine. For instance, information about diet for Afro-Caribbean people should include foods commonly eaten by people from this community. Similarly, Muslim women, for example, must be consulted about the acceptability of certain kinds of information such as abortion, birth control and other health issues, such as HIV/AIDS or breastfeeding.

The process of developing patient information for minority groups will be greatly helped if your (extended) project team includes someone with previous experience of this work or with knowledge of one or more of the translated languages. Contact the Commission for Racial Equality to identify local groups in your area (*see* Useful contacts, p 103).

Access to an interpreter may be preferred by some people to translated versions of an information package (*see* the Information point opposite).

 Action points

- Think about the need to translate information into other languages (even where English is understood) when you start work. Remember to include questionnaires, consent forms, posters and other documentation that you may require later on in the project.
- Find out about and consider any cultural differences that may influence the content of your material.
- Determine which groups you need to cater for and what other materials are already in use. Remember that different needs, levels of literacy and dialects can exist within the same language group. It is helpful if the translator speaks the same dialect as the target group and is of the same gender (where appropriate).

- Identify gaps in existing information and areas where certain ethnic and religious groups have different needs from the wider community (for example, sickle-cell anaemia is more prevalent among some black West Indian and other groups).
- Use appropriate images of people from different ethnic groups in all material.
- Translation can be expensive, so get estimates from a number of sources before the work begins. You will also need specialist typesetters for languages that use a different alphabet. Ask translators for samples of previous work and approach people who have previously used these translation services for advice. You may be able to save money by collaborating with other organisations that translate material (for example, health authorities and trusts) and/or by producing multi-lingual literature (that is, one leaflet printed in more than one language).
- It is recommended that 'back' translation is conducted on all health resources. This means that a second translator translates the final draft back into English to check that the meaning is correct. Ask a person with no prior familiarity with the publication to proofread translated texts for spelling errors and typing mistakes.

Further reading

Adams K (2002). 'Making the best use of health advocates and interpreters'. *BMJ*, vol 325, pS9.

Conroy SP, Mayberry JF (2001). 'Patient information booklets for Asian patients with ulcerative colitis'. *Public Health*, vol 115, pp 418–20.

Effective Communication with South Asian People Affected with Cancer (2002). Produced by the Black and Ethnic Minority Project at Macmillan Cancer Relief.

In Good Faith (June 2000) is a resource guide for mental and spiritual wellbeing produced by the Mental Health Foundation. It aims to signpost people, potentially from different ethnic backgrounds, to sources of support that are sensitive to the spiritual dimension.

National Information Forum (1998). *How to Provide Information Well to Bangladeshi, Chinese, Indian and Pakistani People*. London: National Information Forum.

National Information Forum (2001). *Information for Asylum Seekers and Refugees*. London: National Information Forum.

---

i

- The **Institute of Translation and Interpreting** promotes and develops the science and practice of translation and interpreting and monitors standards of competence and good practice, conduct and ethics. It also produces a directory listing accredited translators and interpreters @ www.iti.org.uk
- **Language Line** and **EITI** provide professionally trained interpreters 24 hours a day, 365 days a year @ www.languageline.co.uk www.eiti.com
- The Department of Health's **Ethnic Minority Health Programme** website provides useful links @ www.doh.gov.uk/minorityhealth
- For an insight into the use of interpreters within public services, contact **INTRAN** (*see* Useful contacts, p 103).
- Many people, including those from ethnic minorities, wish to know about alternative therapies. The **NHS Directory of Complementary and Alternative Medicine (CAM)** provides dedicated easy access listings of all practitioners, who by a process of self-selection, have put themselves forward to work either directly in NHS practices or from their own practice on a referral basis @ www.nhsdirectory.org

---

Reaching people with disabilities

The Disability Discrimination Act 1995 (DDA) introduced new laws and measures aimed at ending the discrimination that many disabled people face. The Act gives disabled people new rights, such as access to facilities and services that are available to members of the public, including hospitals, clinics, doctors' surgeries and pharmacies. Service providers have a duty not to discriminate against disabled people. The duties are:

■ not to refuse service
■ not to provide a worse standard of service
■ not to offer service on worse terms.

Since October 1999, providers of services – whether paid for or free – are required to take reasonable steps to:

■ change a policy, practice, or procedure that makes it impossible, or unreasonably difficult, for disabled people to make use of the service
■ offer an auxiliary aid or service if it would enable (or make it easier for) disabled people to make use of services
■ provide a reasonable alternative method of making services available where a physical feature makes it impossible, or unreasonably difficult, for disabled people to make use of them.

From October 2004, service providers will have to make 'reasonable adjustments' to the physical features of their premises in order to ensure that it is not impossible or unreasonably difficult for disabled people to access the services offered. This will be of particular import to those providing services such as health information resource centres. It will also have an impact on signage. For example, are the information leaflet racks clearly signposted and accessible?

Disabled people are a diverse group with different requirements that service providers need to consider. Service providers have a duty to:

■ produce information in a format such as Braille or on audiotape for blind and partially sighted service users
■ provide a sign-language interpreter
■ take more time to explain to a person with learning difficulties how to take prescribed medicine.

A service provider's duty to make reasonable adjustments is a duty owed to disabled people at large; it is not simply a duty that is weighed up in relation to each individual disabled person who wants to access a service. Service providers should be thinking now about the accessibility of their services to disabled people.

They should anticipate the requirements of disabled people and the adjustments that may have to be made for them. They are expected to consult with disabled users about how to provide services that meet their needs – whether or not they already have disabled users – and should not wait until a disabled person wants to use a service before planning for the reasonable adjustments they need to make.

---

i

■ **DDA Information** has produced a range of information leaflets, including:
  – what service providers need to know
  – some useful suggestions for when you meet disabled people
  – factsheets.
  The DDA publications list is available online @ www.disability.gov.uk
■ **The Disability Rights Commission** provides a wide range of information in an accessible format @ www.drc-gb.org

Further reading

Accessible Health Information (August 2002) is a 70-odd page report that details the findings of a one-year project on the accessibility to disabled people of information provided by the NHS. It relates the experiences and opinions of disabled people in Merseyside who took part in the consultation. Contact: Dr Laurence Clark or Dr Joyce Carter, Central Liverpool NHS Primary Care Trust, Hamilton House, 24 Pall Mall, Liverpool L3 6AL. Tel: 0151 285 2000.

Accessibility Matters. Norfolk guidelines on making information accessible was published in March 2001. A useful guide which covers a number of the issues raised in this section has been producted by Norfolk County Council in association with Norfolk Health Authority (*see* Useful contacts, p 103).

National Information Forum (1999). *Disability Information in Hospitals*. London: National Information Forum. Research study on the benefits of providing basic disability information in hospitals, and the most appropriate way in which it should be provided.

People with visual impairment

Standard written information is often unsuitable for people with visual impairment. There are a number of ways of communicating information to blind and partially sighted people. Printed material may be suitable, particularly when a clear font, large print, spacing, contrast and/or textures are used in its production. For some people, it may be more suitable to receive information aurally. Retention of information given by word of mouth can be enhanced by the use of a dictaphone, or pre-recorded audio cassettes.

Patient information should also be available in Braille – however, only about one in five blind or partially sighted people can use Braille. The Royal National Institute of the Blind (RNIB) can be contacted for further advice on producing material for people who are visually impaired. It has an extensive Braille library and can find out whether a document is already available in Braille (*see* Useful contacts, p 103).

Social services has a duty to provide rehabilitation services, and may be contacted for information on services available in a particular area.

The DDA Code of Practice states the following list of auxiliary aids or services that 'it might be reasonable' to provide, to ensure that services are accessible to people with visual impairments:

- readers
- documents in large or clear print, Moon (a rarely-used embossed font using the standard alphabet) or Braille
- information on computer diskette
- information on audiotape
- telephone services to supplement other information
- spoken announcements or verbal communication
- accessible websites
- assistance with guiding
- audio description services
- large print or tactile maps/plans and three-dimensional models
- touch facilities.

> **i**
>
> - **The RNIB Helpline** on 0845 7669999 can give help on producing information in alternative formats such as Braille and audiotape, as well as details of services available @ www.rnib.org.uk/seeitright provides details of their series of 12 information leaflets
> - **BETSIE** (BBC Education Text to Speech Internet Enhancer) is a simple programming language that is intended to alleviate some of the problems experienced by people using text-to-speech systems for web browsing @ www.bbc.co.uk/education/betsie/about.html
> - **The National Library for the Blind** website @ www.nlbuk.org provides an online catalogue that lists publications for the visually impaired. Use the keyword search facility to determine whether resources exist in the area you wish.
> - **Bobby** is an internet tool that was created to help web page authors identify and repair barriers to access by individuals with disabilities. Bobby tests web pages using the guidelines established by the World Wide Web Consortium's Web Access Initiative @ www.w3.org/WAI. For more information on Bobby, and how to test the accessibilty of your site, go to 'About' @ http://bobby.watchfire.com

People with hearing impairment

People who are deaf or hard of hearing may communicate using sign language, lip-reading, written English or a combination of these. British Sign Language (BSL) is often the first language of people who have been deaf from early in life, with English as their second language. People who have become deaf later in life (often termed 'deafened') are more likely to lip-read and have a better understanding of English. People who become deaf after middle age may find it difficult to learn BSL. Consider using a sign language video, including subtitles, to develop health information for deaf people. Contact the Royal National Institute for Deaf People (RNID) for further information (*see* Useful contacts, p 103).

The DDA Code of Practice states the following list of auxiliary aids or services that 'it might be reasonable' to provide to ensure that services are accessible to people with hearing disabilities:

- written information (such as a leaflet or guide)
- a facility for taking and exchanging written notes
- a verbatim speech-to-text transcription service
- non-permanent induction loop systems
- subtitles
- videos with sign language interpretation
- information displayed on a computer screen
- accessible websites
- textphones, telephone amplifiers and inductive couplers
- teletext displays
- audiovisual telephones
- qualified sign language interpreters or lipspeakers.

Video interpreting

> **@**
>
> Available at:
> www.rnid.org.uk/html/
> information/technology/
> video_interpreting/
> home.htm

The RNID has developed a video interpreting service and is setting up test sites in public access areas across the country. The service has been developed to help combat the shortage of sign language interpreters by making their service available over a video phone. The service is not intended as a replacement for face-to face interpreting support, but can be used for meetings that are arranged at short notice, one-to-one and/or less than 30 minutes long.

> **i**
>
> The Doctor Patient Partnership campaign, entitled 'Are you sure your patients hear what you have to say?', provides tips for GPs and other health care professionals on how to communicate more effectively with deaf and hard of hearing patients @ www.dpp.org.uk

People with learning difficulties

Professionals often overlook the particular need of people with learning difficulties for good quality information. People in this group sometimes say that clinical staff do not treat them as ordinary adults and seem to think they are suffering from mental illness. Some of this group are unable to read but do understand clear signs and pictorial information. Try to involve some of them in your consultation exercise, or consult organisations that represent them.

Books Beyond Words actively address the problems of understanding that people with learning and communications difficulties experience. The stories are told through colour pictures, helping readers to cope with events such as going to the doctor, bereavement, sexual abuse and depression. The stylised drawings include mime and body language to communicate simple, explicit messages to the reader.

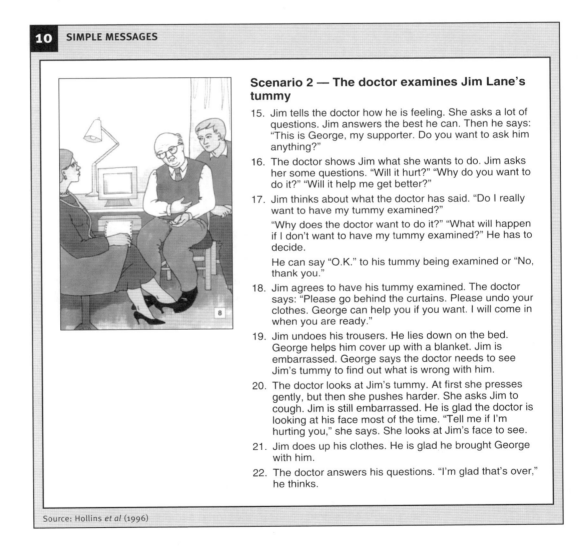

10 SIMPLE MESSAGES

Scenario 2 — The doctor examines Jim Lane's tummy

15. Jim tells the doctor how he is feeling. She asks a lot of questions. Jim answers the best he can. Then he says: "This is George, my supporter. Do you want to ask him anything?"

16. The doctor shows Jim what she wants to do. Jim asks her some questions. "Will it hurt?" "Why do you want to do it?" "Will it help me get better?"

17. Jim thinks about what the doctor has said. "Do I really want to have my tummy examined?"

    "Why does the doctor want to do it?" "What will happen if I don't want to have my tummy examined?" He has to decide.

    He can say "O.K." to his tummy being examined or "No, thank you."

18. Jim agrees to have his tummy examined. The doctor says: "Please go behind the curtains. Please undo your clothes. George can help you if you want. I will come in when you are ready."

19. Jim undoes his trousers. He lies down on the bed. George helps him cover up with a blanket. Jim is embarrassed. George says the doctor needs to see Jim's tummy to find out what is wrong with him.

20. The doctor looks at Jim's tummy. At first she presses gently, but then she pushes harder. She asks Jim to cough. Jim is still embarrassed. He is glad the doctor is looking at his face most of the time. "Tell me if I'm hurting you," she says. She looks at Jim's face to see.

21. Jim does up his clothes. He is glad he brought George with him.

22. The doctor answers his questions. "I'm glad that's over," he thinks.

Source: Hollins *et al* (1996)

 Action points

- Contact specialist organisations (such as those provided in the Information point, overleaf), for advice about the needs of the groups they represent and about the kind of health information that is already in existence.
- Send for information to find out your duties under the Disability Discrimination Act 1995.
- Include people with disabilities and other special needs, and the groups that support and represent them, in your patient consultation exercises.

> *i*
>
> - **People First** is an organisation that helps people with learning difficulties speak up for themselves, with help and support if needed @ www.peoplefirst.org.uk
> - **Plain Facts** is a magazine about research for people with learning difficulties and their supporters produced at the Norah Fry Research Centre. Each issue of Plain Facts is about the findings of a different research project.
> - **Makaton** is a unique language programme offering a structured, multi-modal approach for the teaching of communication, language and literacy skills. Devised for children and adults with a variety of communication and learning disabilities, Makaton is used extensively throughout the UK and has been adapted for use in over 40 other countries @ www.makaton.org
> - **Change** is a national charity run by disabled people. It campaigns for the rights of learning disabled people, especially people with learning disabilities who are deaf or blind. They produce a set of three women's health booklets on depression, planning a baby and the contraceptive Depo-Provera.
> - **The Elfrida Society** is another useful source of information on accessible health leaflets for people with learning difficulties @ www.elfrida.com
> - **Mencap** @ www.mencap.org.uk/html/services/accessibility_services.htm provides documents about making information more accessible to people with learning difficulties. Some of its materials relate to communication in general, covering issues such as how to write and design for this audience. Others are related to how to make websites more accessible for this group.

Further reading

Department of Health (2001). *Valuing People: A new strategy for learning disability for the 21st century*. London: The Stationery Office. White paper setting out a challenging programme of action for improving services @ www.doh.gov.uk/learningdisabilities/strategy.htm

Hollins S, Bernal J, Gregory M (1996). *Going to the Doctor*. Royal College of Psychiatrists/ St George's Hospital Medical School: Books Beyond Words. From the Books Beyond Words series for people with learning difficulties.

A look at the media available

This section highlights some of the special characteristics of each medium. The information points identify specialist sources of advice on detailed technical aspects of production.

Written information

The following factors may influence a decision to produce written information:

- It is usually the cheapest medium and requires less specialist technical expertise to produce in the first instance. (Though this does not mean that everyone can write clearly!)
- Information can be produced to meet the specific needs of very small or very large numbers of patients.
- Patients can have their own copy to take away, carry about all the time, and refer to as and when they want.
- Written information can be readily revised and updated.
- Published information is easily stored and distributed.

Written information must be simple and accessible to patients. One secret of good written communication is having a very clear sense of who you are talking to and what you want to say to them. Just as your style of speaking varies according to who you are talking to, your style of writing needs to vary for different audiences (*see* Choosing your writing style, p 52). As mentioned in Section 5, design is also of key importance.

Visual material

Information in any medium can benefit from the use of visual images, including photos, line drawings, charts and diagrams. The following factors may persuade you to use illustrations:

- They can simplify complex information, inform and entertain.
- They break up large areas of text or speech and make the information less daunting.
- Statistical information is easier to understand in the form of tables, histograms or pie charts.
- Flow diagrams, decision trees and journey maps (*see* Figure 11) help patients to recognise where they are in the processes. (Flow trees are flow diagrams that illustrate the stages people go through when they are making decisions.)

However, do not go overboard. Do you really need a picture of a telephone next to a telephone number in your leaflet? Is there anyone reading it who does not know what a telephone looks like?

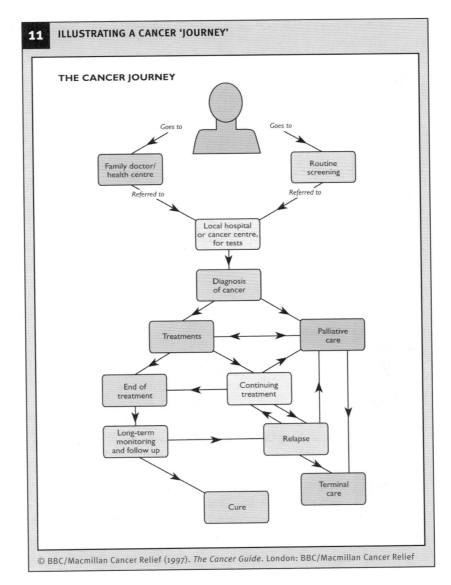

11   **ILLUSTRATING A CANCER 'JOURNEY'**

THE CANCER JOURNEY

© BBC/Macmillan Cancer Relief (1997). *The Cancer Guide*. London: BBC/Macmillan Cancer Relief

Cartoons and animation

Cartoons and animations (moving cartoons and pictures used in video and multimedia) are a valuable tool in various media, for the following reasons:

- A stylised representation is often more acceptable than a picture of the real thing. Patients may be squeamish about a medical 'cutaway' diagram (for example, of the heart). Patients often prefer animation to real medical footage, especially for invasive tests such as inserting a catheter.
- Cartoons can work well in helping people make decisions.
- Animation can be very useful in explaining difficult concepts such as the prevalence of a condition or the relative risks of side effects.
- Moving pictures are useful for anatomy lessons (in, for example, how body parts work) because they give a more accurate presentation than a static picture. For animation and static images, show enough of the body around the part you are illustrating for patients to locate it.
- Cartoons can successfully introduce a lighter tone to the information. However, not all styles of cartoon are the same, and not everyone has the same sense of humour, so be cautious.

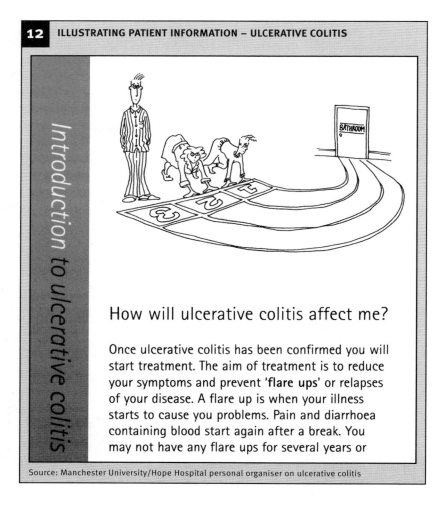

12   ILLUSTRATING PATIENT INFORMATION – ULCERATIVE COLITIS

Introduction to ulcerative colitis

How will ulcerative colitis affect me?

Once ulcerative colitis has been confirmed you will start treatment. The aim of treatment is to reduce your symptoms and prevent 'flare ups' or relapses of your disease. A flare up is when your illness starts to cause you problems. Pain and diarrhoea containing blood start again after a break. You may not have any flare ups for several years or

Source: Manchester University/Hope Hospital personal organiser on ulcerative colitis

> There are many sources for images, but be aware of copyright issues and costs. It is important to include the month and year of printing (and if possible, a review date) on all published material including visuals.
>
> Some examples that specialise in the health field include:
>
> - **The Wellcome Trust Medical Photographic Library** – claims to be the world's leading source of images on the history of medicine, modern biomedical science and clinical medicine, containing over 160,000 images, representing imaging professionals from the UK's leading research laboratories and teaching hospitals @ http://medphoto.wellcome.ac.uk
> - **3DClinic** – produced by BodyOnline, this covers nine body systems, more than 100 healthy body animations and 40 common diseases @ www.bodyonline.co.uk
> - **Mediscan** – has a collection of over 1 million images and 2,000 hours of broadcast quality film footage @ www.mediscan.co.uk

Action points

- Make sure diagrams and photographs are representative of, and understood by, all your patients.
- Keep illustrations simple, including your cover design.
- Make sure a cover illustration represents the topic sensitively and encourages users to explore further.
- If the information is directed at young people, use images of young people.
- Use images of the correct ethnic groups if they will be part of your audience.
- Keep maps simple. For example, show the location of the hospital in relation to important landmarks. Do not attempt to show details unless the map is produced in a large format.
- Avoid information that might change in a few months, such as train or bus times.
- Show patients where they are along the care pathway.
- Take care with humour.
- Test the use of all illustrations with a range of potential users.
- If you are thinking of using recognisable photographs or pictures of real people, make sure that they sign a disclaimer in which they agree not to have any ownership of your material. Model release forms can be obtained from the British Association of Picture Libraries and Agencies (*see* Useful contacts, p 103).

Audio

Audio information could include producing an audio cassette or setting up a telephone line with a recorded message.

Consider the following criteria when you are deciding whether to produce information in an audio medium:

- People who have low levels of literacy can benefit from audio. The Basic Skills Agency estimates that 20 per cent of the adult UK population (around 8 million people) have difficulty with reading.
- Audio information can be offered in different languages to people who may not read in their first spoken language.
- Audio information is suitable for people who are visually impaired.
- All audio information is potentially available to patients in their own home.
- The equipment needed to listen to an audio cassette is not expensive and is widely available. For example, most homes have a telephone.
- Audio cassettes can be used for dramatised examples of different scenarios (for example, a doctor-and-patient encounter).

Action point

- Producing audio material requires a variety of technical expertise and resources. Written material cannot simply be directly recorded because the flow of information alters between the written and spoken word. Some information will have to be rewritten and the order of information reconsidered (this is often called resequencing). A script will need to be written from which audio material can be read.

---

i

- **The RNIB** provides details of organisations that undertake recording work. Tel: 0845 7023153.
- **The Department of Health** runs 21 telephone helplines, including NHS Direct @ www.doh.gov.uk/phone.htm
- **NHS24**, the equivalent to NHSDirect in Scotland, may be able to help @ www.nhs24.scot.nhs.uk.
- **The Telephone Helplines Association** produces a directory including more than 1,000 national, regional and local telephone helplines throughout England, Wales, Scotland and Northern Ireland that follow principles of good practice @ www.helplines.org.uk

---

Case study: The College of Health's 'Healthline' tape service

The College of Health has produced audiotapes on over 500 health-related topics since 1984. These tapes are available under licence and are an inexpensive way of improving and expanding services that health information providers offer to clients. The tapes are designed to be listened to on the phone and offer a simple way of providing health information at home 24 hours a day, 365 days a year. The tapes are professionally produced and the information is regularly updated and validated by medical experts.

Healthline is available to subscribers of *Candis* magazine, *Health Which?* and in factsheet format to Which Online. It is also available in Hull, where the tape directory is printed in the local phone book, receiving more than 200,000 calls a year.

Healthline is also licensed to NHS Direct Online, where a number of audio clips are available in English and minority ethnic languages, including Cantonese, Punjabi, Gujarati, Urdu and Hindi, as well as Bengali Sylheti dialect.

Video

Broadcast-quality videos should be produced by people with the relevant technical skills, including scripting, storyboarding, filming, lighting, sound recording, video graphics and editing, and are often expensive to produce. Digital video still requires technical skill but is less expensive and a cheaper option if disseminated via websites (*see* DIPEx in the Information point opposite). Local colleges that run media courses may be able to make videos at minimal cost, as practical experience for their students. Videos could possibly be offered in outpatients or in pre-operative packages for a returnable deposit. However, unless the budget is large, a video is unlikely to be a suitable medium for producing information that is to be given to individual patients to take away and keep, so you will probably need to produce a patients' leaflet to complement it in any case.

Video is especially useful for:

- demonstrating a skill that needs to be acquired, such as physical exercises
- expressing emotions

- showing other people talking about their experience of medical conditions
- stimulating discussion among a group of patients and carers.

If patients themselves are to be included in a video you are making, you must obtain their consent in writing and they must be aware who may see the video (*see* Legal liability, p 15).

Case study: Patient demand for video

Our 'information for patients research group' conducted a formal study in which 300 patients were asked which educational tool would help them most to understand more about their cancer diagnosis and empower them to become more involved in decision-making. 89 per cent indicated that an information video would be helpful and 87 per cent had easy access to a video player.

Source: Macmillan Consultant Clinical Oncologist, Addenbrooke's Hospital, Cambridge and The Primrose Oncology Centre, Bedford

---

i

- **Videos for Patients** has produced over 40 patient information videos using celebrities such as John Cleese and Dr Robert Buckman (*see* Useful contacts, p 103).
- **The BMA Library** runs a film and video service (for their members) with titles suitable for patients and the general public (*see* Useful contacts, p 103).
- **Focus TV (FTV Ltd)** delivers a TV-messaging service, which provides health and local news items, to waiting areas in NHS trust settings (*see* Useful contacts, p 103).
- **Discovery Health** is a dedicated health channel @ www.discoveryhealth.co.uk *Also see* The internet, p 77 or Interactive Digital Television (iDTV), p 79.
- **The Database of Individual Patient Experience (DIPEx)** provides video accounts of people relating their experiences of a small series of illness and the impact it has had on their lives @ www.dipex.org

Further reading

Eiser JR, Eiser C (1996). 'Effectiveness of video for health education: a review'. London: Health Education Authority. Recommendations for commissioning video-based interventions and examples of well planned and well evaluated projects.

Multimedia

It can be difficult to distinguish clear boundaries when discussing digital content. Multimedia information can be delivered in a variety of channels, including:

- CD Roms
- DVDs
- standalone touchscreen kiosks
- the internet
- smart cards
- mobile phones.

Multimedia (a combination of text, audio, video and visuals contained with a computer program) enables you to deliver information in a wide variety of ways within a single package. To be useful, a multimedia programme should offer patients something they cannot get from other sources (such as information leaflets). The principal advantage of multimedia is that it allows the patient to actually interact with the programme.

Multimedia offers the following benefits:

- If it is developed properly, users can choose between different ways of learning – through text, sound, symbols and animation.
- Patients can control the way they access the programme, with some people choosing to follow it in a linear manner and others jumping around according to their area of immediate interest and concern. They may also choose to replay sections of the presentation.
- Multimedia is especially suitable for children who may be reluctant to read printed information about their condition, or be unable to do so. An interactive computer programme is a child-friendly medium that is likely to encourage them to learn about their condition and find out about treatments.
- Multimedia packages can easily facilitate the collection of user feedback. This is done with an internal audit system (often referred to as the 'black box', the nickname given to aircraft flight recorders) that logs which screens are viewed – and which are not – and for how long. They may also pose questions to patients within the programme. This provides insights into the patient's learning process, which can be fed back into the development cycle.
- Some systems accept input of individual patient data, such as age, gender and symptoms. (This was a feature of one of the pioneering systems, developed by Wennberg and Mulley at the Foundation for Informed Medical Decision Making in the United States, now known as Health Dialog.) In this kind of system, the decision-analysis software processes these data and helps to identify treatment options that are applicable to the particular patient. This information can then be printed out for both the patient and the clinician.

A number of factors needs to be taken into account in reaching a decision about presenting information using multimedia:

- It can be very costly and requires specific IT skills, as well as professional graphic design expertise.
- Many patients will not have encountered multimedia before and may be unfamiliar with its capabilities and nervous of using it. They will need to be shown what it can do.
- Few people like reading lots of text on screen.
- Children are likely to find multimedia easier and more exciting to use than older people who may be less familiar with the technology.
- You will need advice in assessing how easy it is to update content within the multimedia package. Can it be linked to the internet or integrated with other systems? How long will the equipment last before needing an upgrade and what will this cost?
- You will need to think about how you will distribute, and provide technical support for, such a product, especially if users will be expected to have a fairly up-to-date computer on which to run it.

---

i

People with a specific interest in this area may wish to contact the Electronic Publishing Specialist Group @ www.epsg.org.uk which looks at desktop publishing, digital imaging, multimedia and the web.

◧ Case study: Castle Hill Hospital colorectal information package

In the development of the colorectal cancer information package by Hull University/Castle Hill Hospital, the patients involved said that they would prefer written material but when they were shown a computerised version of the information they changed their minds. They liked the flexibility to choose which information to view, in whichever manner they liked, as well as the ability to move through the package at their own pace. The developers went on to produce a multimedia version, which was used as a template for other specialties within the hospital, such as breast cancer.

CD Roms

Experience from the Promoting Patient Choice sites showed that although CD Roms were initially popular, they never really took off as much as expected. Updating them is not that easy and many disks are formatted for PCs only, so that Apple Mac users cannot read them. Today it's more popular to produce stuff for the web as it's accessible to a wider range of people – and it's easier to update.

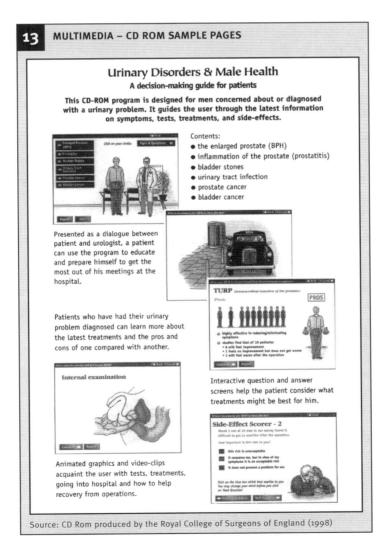

13 MULTIMEDIA – CD ROM SAMPLE PAGES

Urinary Disorders & Male Health
A decision-making guide for patients

This CD-ROM program is designed for men concerned about or diagnosed with a urinary problem. It guides the user through the latest information on symptoms, tests, treatments, and side-effects.

Contents:
- the enlarged prostate (BPH)
- inflammation of the prostate (prostatitis)
- bladder stones
- urinary tract infection
- prostate cancer
- bladder cancer

Presented as a dialogue between patient and urologist, a patient can use the program to educate and prepare himself to get the most out of his meetings at the hospital.

Patients who have had their urinary problem diagnosed can learn more about the latest treatments and the pros and cons of one compared with another.

Interactive question and answer screens help the patient consider what treatments might be best for him.

Animated graphics and video-clips acquaint the user with tests, treatments, going into hospital and how to help recovery from operations.

Source: CD Rom produced by the Royal College of Surgeons of England (1998)

@ www.interactiveeurohealth.com

@ www.showme.uk.com

@ www.med-it.co.uk

For some samples of successful CD Roms produced in the health care field, see:

- **Interactive Euro Health** – CD Roms on asthma, diabetes and cardiovascular disease
- **Show me** – a project that produced a CD Rom about bedwetting. Now produces content for NHS Direct, and Health Development Agency
- **Med-it** – another King's Fund project (Bristol Urge incontinence) now producing a range of resources for different channels
- *Urinary Disorders and Male Health – A decision-making guide for patients* is a CD Rom developed by the Royal College of Surgeons, the British Association of Urological Surgeons and Merck Sharp & Dohme (*see* Fig 13, opposite).

Kiosks

@ www.intouchwithhealth.co.uk
www.jsc.co.uk/medibook.htm
www.starthere.org

A number of organisations develop health information for delivery via kiosks. These can be placed in foyers of hospitals and other public buildings such as libraries and train stations, and are often accessed using touch screens, which remove the need for a mouse or keyboard. Some also have print-out facilities so that users can take copies of the information away with them.

@ www.nhsdirect.nhs.uk
(click on *About NHS Direct*)

NHS Direct has developed and distributed about 200 'Information Points' – computer kiosks that provide free access to the health advice and information available on the NHS Direct Online website.

Further reading

Some research on kiosks for consumer health information has been conducted by City University @ www-digitalhealth.soi.city.ac.uk/isrg/dohabstracts.htm

A survey of health information on electronic public information systems (HEA/SPIN 1999) is available from SPIN @ www.spin.org.uk

Jones RB, Balfour F, Gillies M, Stobo D, Cawsey AJ, Donaldson K (2001). 'The accessibility of computer-based health information for patients: kiosks and the web'. *Medinfo*, vol 10, pp 1469–73.

The following are considered the 'pioneering' papers in the use of kiosks, and are still useful today:

Jones RB, Edgerton E, Baxter I *et al* (1993). 'Where should a public access health information system be sited?' *Interacting with Computers*, vol 5, pp 413–21

Jones RB, Navin LM, Murray KJ (1993). 'Use of a community-based touch-screen public-access health information system'. *Health Bulletin*, vol 51, pp 34–42.

Awards

A number of organisations provide awards for the production of multimedia (*see* Useful contacts, p 103). These include:

@ www.healthcare-computing.co.uk/hitea/aboutawards.htm

- **The British Computer Society (BCS)** – the chartered institution for professionals working in all aspects of information technology and information systems engineering. Has a number of health-related informatic sub-groups that will be of interest to people developing digital patient information.

- **The British Interactive Multimedia Association (BIMA)** – the trade association for companies and individuals involved in the interactive media sector in the UK.
- **CTIC Medicine (Computers in Teaching Initiative)** – develops computer systems for training pre- and post-graduate health care professionals.
- A number of awards also exist for health websites (*see the Information point overleaf*).

---

i

- **Lis-medical** is an open discussion list for members of this UK medical and health care library @ lis-medical@jiscmail.ac.uk
- **Consumer Health Informatics** is for anyone developing or evaluating electronic methods for the direct use of patients and the public. This includes patient education, information about services and other sources of help, and computer–patient interviewing @ consumer-health-informatics@jiscmail.ac.uk
- **con-healthinc** is a discussion forum for members of the Consumer Health Information Consortium (CHIC) and others with a professional interest in consumer/patient information to exchange information @ con-health@mailbase.ac.uk
- **The Foundation for Informed Medical Decision-Making** was the original developer of patient resources that allow the physician and the patient to select a treatment that reflects the values and preferences of the patient as well as important clinical considerations. See under 'Relationships' @ www.healthdialog.com
- The US-based **Science Panel on Interactive Communication and Health (SciPICH)** examined interactive health communication (IHC) technology and its potential impact on the health of the public (April 1999).See under 'Publications' @ www.health.gov/scipich/pubs/finalreport.htm
- **Society of Public Information Networks (SPIN)** has more than 300 members, including local authorities, health agencies, libraries, museums, central government departments, voluntary organisations and private sector companies. All are involved in disseminating or exchanging information with the public and staff within their own organisations (*see* Useful contacts, p 103).

Further reading

Kasper JF, Mulley AG, Wennberg JE (1992). 'Developing shared decision-making programs to improve the quality of health care'. *Quality Review Bulletin*, vol 18, pp 183–90.

Leonard J (1994). *Interacting: Multimedia and health*. London: Health Education Authority.

The internet

The web is so vast, and the people's desire to use it to search for health information ever expanding, that a dedicated publication is necessary to cover the topic (*see* Further reading, p 81). However, as a starting point, *see* Useful websites (p 117).

One of the first, and most often-repeated, suggestions for inclusion in this second edition of the guide was for guidance on how to put patient information on to a website. The following information and views are provided by Colon Cancer Concern:

> It is well worth considering having your patient information accessible through your website because the more you have on your site, the greater its potential use. Utilising the website in this way also enables you to widen access to your information and to raise your profile – as many hospitals and voluntary organisations have already discovered.
>
> When transferring information onto your website, you should consider whether to simply copy and adapt your existing information or start again, by using the available technology. For example, it is now possible to enhance documents with a supporting A–Z and to add animation to diagrams. Whichever route you take will depend on who is building your site and how much money is available.
>
> The quickest and cheapest way to include patient information is by adding pages of text to your site. This makes it easy for you to update or alter the site whenever you

wish. However, it also means that anyone viewing your page can download, manipulate or change the text without your knowledge or permission. You also have no control over how the page appears on an individual computer screen.

One alternative is to use Adobe's Acrobat software to produce pdfs. While this means an initial expense in purchasing the software, it is worth considering. Because the information is put on the site as a complete image, it cannot be tampered with: when it is printed off, it will appear exactly as it was designed. Be careful of using elaborate text or graphics, however, as they will increase the time that pages take to appear on screen, and you could lose people who are not prepared to wait.

> @
> www.adobe.com

If you use Acrobat, it is advisable to add a link to the site where a version of the program can be downloaded free of charge. This will enable people to read the documents.

There are some drawbacks to placing information on your site. You have no way of gauging if the information you provide is fulfilling a person's needs and it cannot be tailored to an individual or adapted for specific cases. There are ways of asking for personal details before allowing a download, but you may not want to put obstacles in the way of those wanting information. Also, it is a cold form of communication, in as much as it doesn't enable you to establish and build personal relationships with potential supporters.

Cancer Colon Concern (2002)

---

i

- If you are unfamiliar with the Internet, visit **BBC WebWise** @ www.bbc.co.uk/webwise
  Alternatively, contact learndirect for details of an internet course that can be taken at home or from one of the learndirect centres @ www.learndirect.co.uk/personal Tel: 0800 101901.
- **Popular Communication** @ www.popcomm.co.uk co-ordinates the Charity and Public Service Publishing Awards. One of the categories is for websites, and health-oriented sites have often been finalists in this category. In 2001 the winner was the Royal National Institute for the Deaf.
- Details of numerous awards for health websites can be found on the internet. One of the most appropriate is the **BMA Patient Information Website Award** @ www.bma.org.uk/ap.nsf/Content/LIBBMAPatient InformationAward#app 2
- For details of making websites accessible to people with disabilities, see **'Bobby'** in the Information point, p 66.
- **The European Commission** published its long-awaited policy document on quality criteria for health websites on 7 December 2002, entitled *eEurope 2002: quality criteria for health related websites* @ www.jmir.org/2002/3/e15/ index.htm. The document is based on a series of meetings held during 2001 and drew together key players from government departments, international organisations, non-governmental organisation and industry, to explore current practices and experiments in this field.

For more website listings, *see* Useful websites, p 117.

New technologies

> @
> www.doh.gov.uk/ebusiness
> _dhmain/ebusiness.pdf

The Department of Health published its e-Business Strategy in September 2001. It refers to a range of services and is a useful summary of some of the many projects currently being undertaken. It makes specific reference to good quality patient information:

Citizens will have the assurance when they access e-services, eg NHS Direct, that the content of material is good quality. Health guidelines will be provided by the National Institute for Clinical Excellence...

Department of Health (2001)

As part of the Government's look at new technologies, a couple of services have been trialled, and in some cases implemented, with Interactive Digital Television (iDTV) and Bedside TV.

Interactive Digital Television (iDTV)

In early 2001, the Department of Health awarded four companies (DKTV Ltd, Communicopia Productions Ltd, Channel Health and Flextech Telewest – *Living Health*) funding to pilot various strands of an iDTV health offering.

The pilot projects explored a range of transactional services, such as booking an appointment, seeing an NHS Direct nurse on TV and providing a reminder service on TV.

The Department has announced that a programme of work will focus on developing a version of NHS Direct for digital TV and to make it available nationwide. Working with commercial partners from the media and broadcasting industries, the Department of Health and the NHS will develop a service that will enable people to have easy and fast access at home to trusted information and advice on health, healthcare and the NHS. Such a service will complement the NHS Direct telephone helpline and NHS Direct Online website.

They will continue to examine the more interactive uses of digital TV, perhaps including applications such as ordering a repeat prescription, requesting more information about a local service and networking through the TV with others who have similar health problems or conditions. Some of these transactional services, if successful, will be considered for inclusion in the NHS Direct digital TV service.

An independent evaluation of the pilots has been conducted by City University, London, and by Sheffield University, which provides valuable insights into the feasibility of such services, the likely take-up, the characteristics of users and their patterns of usage, users' perceptions, the impact on these users, and the impact on the NHS.

◼ Case study: Living Health

Living Health is an interactive digital television (iDTV) channel, launched in Birmingham on Telewest Active Digital in June 2001. It has information modules on news, healthy living, men's health, women's health, children's health, illnesses and treatments and local services. It has also introduced two transactional services: GP appointment booking and nurse consultation on the television (inVision).

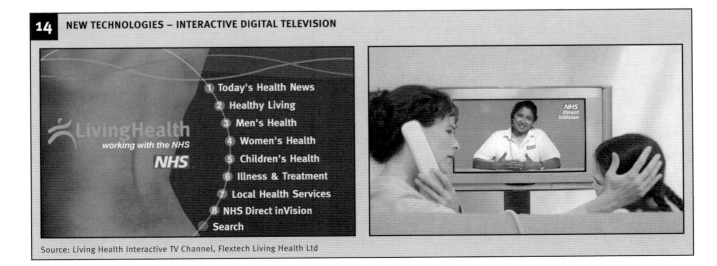

14   **NEW TECHNOLOGIES – INTERACTIVE DIGITAL TELEVISION**

1 Today's Health News
2 Healthy Living
3 Men's Health
4 Women's Health
5 Children's Health
6 Illness & Treatment
7 Local Health Services
8 NHS Direct inVision
Search

LivingHealth working with the NHS *NHS*

NHS Direct inVision

Source: Living Health Interactive TV Channel, Flextech Living Health Ltd

After running the service for a year, conclusions were that there was a proven need for this type of information provision, and that it supported existing primary care organisations. People trusted the information provided because of Living Health's co-branding with the NHS (all information was accredited by Centre for Health Information Quality), and also because the television is a trusted medium. The introduction of transactional services not only demonstrated positive take-up of these services (leading to a feeling of greater empowerment) but they encouraged utilisation of the information service.

Flextech Living Health Ltd

---

i

- **Factor V** is a consultancy involved in both iDTV (with Channel Health) and Bedside TV initiatives @ www.factorv.co.uk
- **Eden Communications** is a consultancy interested in e-government and health and involved with the Living Health iDTV pilot @ www.eden-communications.com

Further reading

Dick P (2002). 'Healthy Options – Interactive dTV pilots'. *Electronic Public Information*, April/May, pp 17–18.

Dick P (2001). 'Towards NHS Direct TV'. *British Journal of Healthcare Computing and Information Management*, vol 18, pp 22–24.

Hain T (2001). 'A quality assurance programme for NHS Digital TV services'. *Health Expectations*, vol 4, pp 260–62.

Webdale J (2001). 'Docs on the box'. *New Media Age*, 04/10/01, pp 35–9.

Webdale J (2001). 'Medical advice body adds web to its scope'. *New Media Age*, 16/08/01, p 1.

Bedside television

Sections 4.19 and 4.20 of the NHS Plan promised that bedside televisions and telephones would be available in every major English hospital (defined as having more that 150 beds) by 2004.

@
Full details of the Bedside Communications Systems initiative are available at: www.nhsestates.gov.uk/ patient_environment/ index.asp

Owned by NHS Estates, the Patient Power project states: 'Most of us have TVs and radios and it is now estimated that around 70% of the population have use of a mobile phone – therefore, why should patients not have access to these services when they are admitted to hospital?' The deadline has been moved forward with a view to making these services available in all major hospitals by 2003. The services are reputed to include access to 'approved' patient information via the TV and internet. Some initial discussion has also taken place about an accompanying bedside radio service.

Mobile health information

The use of faster mobile networks, such as third generation (or 3G), promises delivery of a greater volume of multimedia information (such as pictures and video) and allows for 'always-on' connectivity to the internet. A number of resources have been developed that utilise the text messaging or short messaging service (SMS) capability of most current mobile phones.

i

- **Homerton Hospital** is trialling an SMS service to remind people to turn up for appointments and so reduce the number of 'do not attends'.
- **Sweet Talk**, a project at the University of Dundee, aims to keep adolescents with diabetes motivated and interested in their own health. Using SMS text messaging enables the diabetes team to keep in contact with the young people between clinic visits. Young people are also able to write their own motivational messages.
- **NetDoctor** provides a range of services. One sends you a text message reminding women to take their oral contraceptive. Another is a more general service called BabyText, which helps woman to track their baby's developmental milestones during pregnancy.
- **Future Health Bulletin** is an email service covering the use of the Internet and other new technologies in the health sector @ www.headstar.com/futurehealth
- **The BMA Library** offers a 'medical informatics' information service covering a wide range of journals in this field @ www.bma.org.uk/ap.nsf/Content/LIBMedicalInformaticsInformationService
- **The UK Council for Health Informatics Professions (UKCHIP)** is a new body that will set standards and good practice guidelines for information professionals in the health sector @ www.primis.nottingham.ac.uk/ukchip

Further reading

eHealth Horizons, published by the Sowerby Centre for Health Informatics (July 2000), is a vision document looking at a five-to-ten-year horizon on health @ www.doh.gov.uk/ipu/whatnew/ehealthhorizons.pdf

Masys D (2002). 'Effects of current and future information technologies on the health care workforce'. *Health Affairs*, vol 21, pp 33–41. A paper in which Daniel Masys, director of bioinformatics at the University of California, San Diego, argues that future health care workforces could include informationists (a new type of librarian skilled in retrieving information for clinical care), personal health advocates and advisers (who help consumers find out more about their care) and telemedicine practitioners, presenters, and consultants who specialise in delivering health care at a distance @ www.healthaffairs.org/freecontent/v21n5/s8.htm

Neville R, Greene A, McLeod J, Tracy A, Surie J (2002). 'Mobile phone text messaging can help young people manage asthma'. *BMJ*, vol 325, p 600. Reports on more Scottish innovation in using mobile phone text messaging to help young people manage asthma

Public Health and Information and Communications Technologies (ICTs): Tackling health and digital inequalities in the information age, is a report from John Moore's University providing health care professionals with the background they need to exploit new technology (such as the Internet, mobile phones and digital TV) to improve the public's health. Centre for Public Health, John Moore's University. Tel: 0151 231 4308.

7 Attaining quality

This section looks at some of the initiatives relating to the quality of patient information and how you can utilise them to benchmark your own and others' information. The section concludes with an outline of how to review and pilot your information to ensure it adheres to these standards.

Quality standards

In recent years, much effort has been expended on identifying key standards and criteria for producing and accrediting top quality patient information. A wide range of organisations from every sector have set up numerous quality schemes. Some lay down basic principles for how the editorial process should work to create the information (often called the 'architectural approach'). Others take information that has already been created, and accredit it (the 'archaeological approach'). Some schemes are for certain types of information only – for example, DISCERN is used for information that presents treatment options. Others are applicable only to specific media, such as the internet. Some schemes are fee-based; others are free. The area is a complicated one, and as yet there is no clear 'winner' from the existing schemes.

Quality standards should be universally applicable to all patient resources, irrespective of media. However, some standards, such as navigability and links policies, are particularly relevant to the web:

@
www.equip.nhs.uk

The NHS 'EQUIP' website uses criteria such as navigability and readability to link to sites that will be of interest to UK patient and families. These criteria encapsulate many of the issues considered in many of the quality standards discussed in that section.

- **content** – information contained on the site should be checked by a group of doctors and other experts for quality, accuracy and scope
- **appropriateness** – content should be suitable for the audience
- **design and navigability** – ease of use, speed and appropriate use of graphics is assessed
- **authorship** – authors and those who were involved in creation (for example, any patients who were involved) and level of expertise of authors and reputation of the organisation should be identified. Contact details should be available
- **sponsorship** – sponsors should be clearly stated and suitable
- **readability** – appropriate level of language for audience
- **currency** – date of update should be clear and content still valid
- **legibility** – sites should ideally adhere to RNIB guidelines for the visually impaired and partially sighted
- **accessibility** – there should be no registration, cost or special software required to enter the site, and sites should be viewable in Netscape and Internet Explorer
- **copyright** – the information should be in the public domain.

The US National Cancer Institute has issued exceptional guidance on web design and usability, covering areas such as design considerations and accessibility. This site really says it all, and indeed some of the statements may equally be applied to other forms of information. Its guidance covers the following topics:

@
www.usability.gov/
guidelines

- design process
- design considerations
- content/content organisation
- titles/headings
- page length
- page layout
- font/text size
- reading and scanning
- links
- graphics
- search
- navigation
- software/hardware
- accessibility.

@
www.nhsdirect.nhs.uk/
feedback.asp

NHS Direct Online also has a **Links and Portal Policy**, which, although not currently available online, can be obtained using the feedback form (remember to include a contact email address). This is useful for developers who may be looking to develop their own policies in this area.

A project entitled 'JUDGE', supported by Contact a Family (*see* Useful contacts, p 103), is developing quality standards specifically for websites developed by voluntary health organisations. Their aims are two-fold: first, to help health consumers to make informed decisions about sites, and second, to assist voluntary organisations to produce good quality sites.

Further reading

Anon (1999). 'Health on the Net'. *Health Which?* April, pp 8–11.

Aspects of the NHS Direct patient information service have been evaluated both internally – NHS Direct Online @ www.nhsdirect.nhs.uk/misc/four_year_report.pdf – and independently via Sheffield University and the National Audit Office @ www.shef.ac.uk/uni/academic/R-Z/scharr/mcru/reports.htm and www.nao.gov.uk/publications/vfmsublist/vfm_nhs.htm

The Patient's Internet Handbook (Oct 2001) is written by Robert Kiley and Elizabeth Graham of the Wellcome Trust Library and published by the Royal Society of Medicine @ www.patient-handbook.co.uk

The *Journal of Medical Internet Research* is an international scientific peer-reviewed journal on all aspects of research, information and communication in the health care field using internet and intranet-related technologies @ www.jmir.org/index.htm

He@lth Information on the Internet, from the Royal Society of Medicine, is a bi-monthly newsletter that aims to meet the growing demand from health care professionals for information about health resources available on the internet @ www.hioti.org

The 9 March 2002 *British Medical Journal* (vol 324, issue 7337), was a special theme issue ('Trust me, I'm a website') about evaluating the quality of health information on the internet, and included several key references on the topic. Free online @ http://bmj.com/content/vol324/issue7337

Barnett B (2001). 'Developing a charity Web Site: the experience of Contact a Family'. *He@lth Information on the Internet*; vol 21, pp 4–5.

Childs S (2002a). 'Editorial: Guidelines and resources for designing Web sites'. *He@lth Information on the Internet*, vol 27, pp 1–2.

Childs S (2002b). 'Editorial: How is the Internet used for health information?' *He@lth Information on the Internet*, vol 28, pp 1–2.

Clement WA, Wilson S, Bingham BJ (2002). 'A guide to creating your own patient-oriented website'. *Journal of the Royal Society of Medicine*, vol 95, pp 64–7.

Eysenbach G, Powell J, Kuss O, Sa ER (2002). 'Empirical studies assessing the quality of health information for consumers on the world wide web: a systematic review'. *Journal of the American Medical Association*, vol 287, pp 2691–700.

Jones R (2000). 'Keep ahead of the game if you want to recommend quality Websites to patients. Follow the guide'. *Nursing Standard*, vol 14(44), p 29.

Kiley R (2002). 'Quackery on the Web'. *He@lth Information on the Internet*, vol 15, pp 9–10.

Risk A, Petersen C (2002). 'Health information on the internet: quality issues and international initiatives'. *Journal of the American Medical Association*, vol 287, pp 2713–5.

Shepperd S, Charnock D (2002). 'Against internet exceptionalism'. *BMJ*, vol 324, pp 556–7.

Kitemarking

Another angle to this discussion is that, since the explosion of health information that is available on – and accessed via – the internet, much debate has focused on the value of using kitemarks or trustmarks to assure consumers they can trust the information they are accessing.

The Plain English Campaign charges editing fees for their **Crystal Mark** – an award that ensures clear writing and meaning. It does not assess the accuracy of the content.

@ www.chiq.org/chiq/triangle.htm

The **TriangleMark,** from the Centre for Health Information Quality (CHIQ), aims to offer the public reassurance about all aspects of the quality of health information they are viewing. CHIQ is working with the NHS to explore ways in which the TriangleMark scheme can be adopted nationally.

Royal Colleges and voluntary health organisations may also wish to endorse resources developed around specific conditions. As with Copyright (*see* p 16), the use of logos should be agreed well in advance. Take care to determine what users think of such endorsements.

@ www.jmir.org/2001/4/e28/index.htm

A vast array of other organisations and initiatives are also looking at this area, especially for websites. A report by Ahmad Risk and Joan Dzenowagis (2001) of the World Health Organisation provides a comprehensive review of 13 of the major quality health website standards. It includes eHealth Code of Ethics, Health Internet Ethics, Organizing Medical Networked Information (OMNI), Health on the Net Foundation, URAC, MedCertain and DISCERN. Readers with a particular interest in this area are urged to review this excellent paper. *Also see* Quality standards, p 82.

Conversely, some argue that consumers are not aware of, nor particularly interested in, kitemarking schemes, and that the efforts to develop such are ill founded. A short but effective argument against kitemarking can be found in a *BMJ* editorial (Delamothe 2000).

It has been suggested that a more practical, feasible and acceptable approach than kitemarking involves self-accreditation of health information by the public, in partnership with their health care professional(s). Existing guidelines could be applied to educate consumers to review the following:

- **authorship** – who are the authors, are they qualified to provide the information, and what are their affiliations?
- **attribution** – is the information reliable, and is it referenced?
- **currency** – is the information up to date?
- **disclosure** – who owns/sponsors the information, and do they have a vested interest?
- **audience** – does the information state its intended recipients and target the information accordingly?
- **double check** – use more than one source of information, and where possible in co-operation with health care professionals.

Tools

The King's Fund devised and evaluated the following criteria during its Promoting Patient Choice programme and they still serve as a most useful reminder of the key issues one must consider when producing patient information. The standards were found to be difficult to achieve in their entirety, but represented a 'gold standard' to be aimed for:

The standards found that good quality patient information:

- informs patients about their clinical condition and includes information about all available treatments or management options, including non-intervention
- provides comprehensive and unbiased information about outcomes (risks and benefits) based on systematic reviews of research evidence
- outlines uncertainties and gaps in scientific knowledge
- involves users and professionals in developing and evaluating the materials
- caters for people from a variety of ethnic and cultural backgrounds and for people with learning difficulties
- is regularly reviewed and updated
- is integrated into a planned programme for shared clinical decision-making
- has language and design that are simple and easily understood.

Hi Quality – guidelines on health information quality

Hi Quality was developed by the Centre for Health Information Quality (CHIQ) (*see* organisations below) and is intended to increase awareness about quality assurance issues in relation to health information. The site can be used in two ways – whether you are producing health information and require guidance on how to assure quality standards or are looking for health information and require guidance on how to check its quality (*see* Building on existing information, p 23).

@ www.hiquality.org.uk

DISCERN

DISCERN (Developing an Assessment Instrument for the Clinical Appraisal of Written Consumer Health Information) is a general set of quality criteria established by researchers at the University of Oxford that help consumers and information providers to judge the quality of consumer health information on treatment choices. A handbook has been written to help consumers and producers understand and use DISCERN effectively. It has been written from the patient perspective, but can be used by anyone interested in information about treatment choices (Charnock 1998). All materials are free on the website.

@ www.discern.org.uk

The DISCERN criteria examine the content of the publication rather than how it is provided. They do not address issues about presentation (such as layout, graphics or readability). This is important because a publication may be well presented and readable without being informative and accurate – and vice versa.

DISCERN lists 16 questions to help users and producers of health information to think about quality issues in a systematic way.

- **Qus 1–8** address the reliability of the information and should help you consider whether it can be trusted as a source of information about treatment choices. For example, is it clear which sources were used to compile the publication other than the author or producer?
- **Qus 9–15** focus on specific details of the information relating to patient choices in medical treatment. For example, does your publication describe what would happen if the patient is not treated?
- **Qu 16** is an intuitive summary of the first 15 questions and provides overall ratings of 'high', 'moderate' or 'low'.

The DISCERN criteria can be applied to online information, and users of DISCERN report using the criteria to judge the quality of information in a variety of media, including videos and CDs. Interactive workshops have been developed to train users of health information to apply the DISCERN criteria. The aim of these workshops is to provide an opportunity for interactive learning, and to be a forum for raising awareness about the provision of information to the public.

The DISCERN instrument has also been used as the basis for the development of a number of other quality tools, which focus on particular conditions or audiences – TriLET and EQIP (below) are two such examples.

Further reading

Charnock D (1998). *The DISCERN Handbook: Quality criteria for consumer health information on treatment choices*. Oxford: Radcliffe Medical Press.

Charnock D, Shepperd S, Needham G, Gann R (1999). 'DISCERN: an instrument for judging the quality of written consumer health information on treatment choices'. *Journal of Epidemiology and Community Health*, vol 53, pp 105–11.

Rees CE, Ford JE, Sheard CE (2002). 'Evaluating the reliability of DISCERN: a tool for assessing the quality of written patient information on treatment choices'. *Patient Education and Counseling*, vol 47, pp 273–5.

Shepperd S, Charnock D (2002) 'A 5 star system for rating the quality of health information based on DISCERN'. *Health Information and Libraries Journal*.

Other tools

TriLET (Trials Leaflet Evaluation Tool)

Researchers at the University of Leicester are developing a tool to define quality standards for information leaflets about clinical trials, and to create a reliable and valid instrument that can be used to assess the extent to which leaflets meet these standards. Guidelines on the production of leaflets for potential research participants have been developed both locally and nationally, but they do not adequately reflect best practice in information production, and may fail to address patients' own priorities for information. In addition, they are unsuitable as a means of appraising quality. TriLET aims to address issues not covered by DISCERN (such as presentation and design) and those that are relevant only to potential research participants.

For further information, email: md11@leicester.ac.uk

Further reading on TriLET

Anon (1999) 'Guidelines for researchers: patient information sheet and consent form'. *Bulletin of Medical Ethics*, vol 148, pp 8–12.

Lees N, Dixon-Woods M, Young B, Heney D, Thornton H (2001). 'CaTLET: Evaluation of information leaflets for patients entering cancer trials (abstract)'. *Psycho-oncology*, vol 10, p 266.

See Information on clinical trials, p 48.

Ensuring Quality Information for Patients (EQIP)

A team at Great Ormond Street Hospital is currently developing a quality assessment tool for patient information. Unlike existing tools such as DISCERN, it is hoped that EQIP will be applicable to all categories of information, including information on conditions, operations, drugs and services. EQIP has been successfully used by the team in an audit setting and can also be used as a checklist for producing high quality information. While it is being developed with the aim of assessing printed literature, its use can also be extended to other media. EQIP is currently being subjected to a rigorous validation procedure, the results of which should be available in 2003.

Email: info@gosh.nhs.uk

SPLASH

Survey of Pharmacy Leaflets – A self-help guide is a quality assessment tool, developed by Health Promotion Wales in 1996 and now published on the web. It aims to enable pharmacists to appraise and choose the most helpful information leaflets to use in their pharmacy. The SPLASH test assesses the key points that ensure a leaflet 'works', holds the reader's attention and is easily understood. It assesses the content of leaflets, how they are written and how well they have been designed and illustrated. A new edition is planned for 2003.

www.hpw.wales.gov.uk/ tools/splash/index.html

QUICK (QUality Information ChecKlist)

This is a UK website designed to help children and young people assess the quality of the information they find on the Internet, with the necessary tools to decide whether or not a site is giving them useful information. Offers quizzes, puzzles and a chance to pit their wits against Cyberquack.

www.quick.org.uk

Organisations

Centre for Health Information Quality (CHIQ)

The Centre for Health Information Quality (CHIQ) was established in 1997 by the Department of Health, as part of an independent charity called the Help for Health Trust. CHIQ works with a range of health organisations to maximise public confidence in health information. It achieves this by providing training and consultancy services, appraisal of health information, and by raising awareness of the quality issues around consumer health information.

CHIQ believes all health information should be developed to be accurate, clear and relevant. In addition, any quality assurance model for a health information service should comprise three phases:

- identification of standards
- training and support for information staff
- service monitoring and feedback.

Training is for producers and providers to gain expertise in the fields of communication and information appraisal. This is especially for information producers working outside the NHS, and for those within NHS PALS, clinical governance and clinical informatics teams. CHIQ offers:

- **consultancy** – available for those with the responsibility to develop or maintain high quality health information services
- **appraisals/accreditation** – expert appraisers review information and related services in any media format (eg leaflets, websites and multimedia resources)
- **online resources** – including Quick and Hi Quality (*see* p 87).

Health Quality Service (HQS)

The Health Quality Service is a not-for-profit organisation based in London. It runs an independent accreditation programme based on quality standards for the practice, organisation and delivery of health care services. It also offers provider organisations an external survey to demonstrate the extent to which they are achieving these standards and awards accreditation to those organisations that demonstrate achievement of all the essential elements.

Section Four of the HQS programme focuses on the patient's experience, with a particular emphasis on the standard of information that patients receive, including the formats in which it is produced and the timeliness of materials being available.

The standards require health care providers to ensure that:

- resources are available for patients, prior to treatment, to help them make informed choices about their condition and treatment options, based on the best available evidence on effective and appropriate interventions
- the materials are written in concise, non-technical language that is easy for people who are not health care professionals to understand and explain:
  - what the procedure involves
  - the treatment alternatives and possible outcomes, together with general and procedure-specific risks
  - possible complications and side effects associated with the surgery or other treatment.
- resources for patients/users and carers promote the concept of shared decision-making
- resources for patients/users and carers are written in concise, plain language, and take account of the needs of particular patient/user groups
- the language and design of resources takes into account the needs of the least able and the less educated
- consideration is given to the production of resources in a range of formats such as large print, or audiotapes, or as may be appropriate for people with learning disabilities, using Makaton symbols and/or pictures
- resources for patients/users are translated into other languages appropriate for the local community and/or the patient/user profile of the hospital/unit.

The above points are assessed by external peer reviewers, who look not only at the resources, but also at their availability, staff awareness of the information and the records of when information is provided to patients/users.

 Action points

- Assess the quality of patient information – both your own and any other that you are considering using. For patient information offering a range of treatment options, the DISCERN instrument can provide this assessment.
- Approach patient information officers and/or audit or quality departments in your own and other organisations – they may have developed guidelines for producing patient information.
- Once you have looked at existing standards, decide which are appropriate for your own material, and apply them accordingly.

Producers of information should be aware that such schemes (or tools), and organisations dedicated to them, do exist.

When it comes to patient resources, and the schemes to produce or appraise them, one size does not fit all. It is the intended audience – your patients – that are the ultimate 'quality standard'. This is why it is so vital to involve patients right from the start in your production of materials (*see* Collecting views of patients and carers, p 35).

Further reading

Nicklin J (2002). 'Improving the quality of written information for patients'. *Nursing Standard*, vol 16(49), pp 39–44.

Shepperd S, Charnock D, Gann B (1999). 'Helping patients access high quality health information'. *BMJ*, vol 319, pp 764–6.

Running a pilot scheme

Once a draft has been produced, it is vital to allow adequate time for consultation and piloting, that is, testing that your information meets its intended aims for its intended audience. Methods are outlined in Section 4. Rushing the work will ultimately affect the quality and acceptability of the finished product. The worst case scenario is that without testing its acceptability beforehand, your product may go unused. Any information you want to use with patients – your own and material produced by other agencies – should be piloted to check:

- whether patients find the information easy or difficult to use
- how well patients have understood the key messages.

Draft patient information packages should be reviewed by:

- **patients you have already consulted, and some new potential users** – there are several ways to do this. You can bring groups together to discuss the draft material or you can send it to the patients and ask them to let you know what they think about the specific aspects of the material, and the material in general. In both cases, ask clear and specific questions and give the following people the chance to say what they think spontaneously:
  - **clinical staff**: within the environment in which they will be used

- **independent experts**: a minimum of two reviewers with expertise in the topic area, who are fully independent of the producers. An independent third party from a voluntary organisation or a professional body may help you to identify suitable people who can be invited to critically appraise the information. Replies from expert reviewers should be anonymous so that they feel free to be honest in their comments (Coulter *et al* 1998).

You will certainly want to ask senior people in your organisation to comment on the draft. The chief executive or director should usually be given a chance to comment. Many trusts with patient information officers have established editorial panels to approve publications.

It is important to give clear guidelines on your draft. If you need to obtain sign off from individuals, then a useful tactic is to include the phrase: 'The deadline for comments is x. It will automatically be assumed that you accept this draft as is, if any communication has not been received by this date.' However, beware of people not receiving the information in time to comment, or indeed, not receiving it at all! Also put a date and version number (eg 12 April 2003, Version 1) on each draft and make sure that everyone is working from the same version.

In addition to showing the importance of piloting material before 'mass' production, the following case study also highlights gaps between patient and professional views on the value of resources (*see* Conflicts of interest, p 42).

◼ Case study: Opposites attract?

A novel way to present information, administered via health visitors, about the different developmental mental health stages for infants from birth to five years, was suggested by project workers at HealthWorks – Dorset's Health Promotion Agency and Poole Primary Care NHS Trust.

Prior to full production, fridge magnets and an accompanying card were piloted with parents and with health care professionals.

Method

A questionnaire, which included the following questions, was administered to 31 of the 53 parents originally given the resources:

- Where have you put the magnet? If it is not on show, why is that?
- Do you like the photograph? What is it that you like/dislike about it?
- Is there anything you would change about it?
- Have you read the attached card? Was it easy to read?
- Was the information on the card useful? If 'yes', why? If 'no', then why not?

Results

These showed that parents:

- generally liked the magnet and its messages
- some did not like the photo it contained
- some did not like the accompanying card for fear of it getting lost.

Health visitors' reactions to continued use of the magnets were mixed. Half felt that something was needed to raise mental health issues but three-quarters questioned the magnet as the correct vehicle for doing this. Concern was also expressed about the time commitment needed.

Conclusions

Before mass production, the following needs should be considered:

- to identify and test a better photo, and find an alternative to the card to provide additional information
- to ensure that health care professionals supported and were willing to disseminate the chosen materials.

 Action points

- Once the first draft is ready, devise a set of multiple choice or short-answer questions.
- Send the draft and questions to a cross-section of the target audience and to clinical experts for comment.
- Also send it to chief executives and clinical directors (where appropriate) for their comments
- Ideally, you should pilot your information in more detail, using some of the techniques mentioned in Collecting views of patients and carers (p 35).

8 Dissemination

This section presents some ways to get your resources known about – if that is what you want. Depending upon your organisational set up, this may be something that is taken care of by people in other departments, for example, in marketing or communications. Even if that is the case, it will be useful to read this section, both for additional ideas and because you will need to consider dissemination when you plan how many copies you will produce. It is also important for you to have thought through not only the production issues, but also how to make sure your material reaches the right place and the right people.

The first question to ask is who comes into contact with your audience. Do you want to circulate your resource only within your own organisation or locality, or do you want to make it available nationally?

Either way, think about how to get the information to health care professionals who work directly with patients. Ideally, some of them will already be aware of your project through your initial exploratory work and piloting, especially if you are working at local level.

- Ask them to discuss the material with you and to think about ways they can make sure that it is given to the people it is intended for. This personal contact with individuals is almost always appreciated.
- Make sure they have enough copies to give out and that they are kept in a place where they won't be forgotten or lost.
- Give them details of how to contact you if they, or the patients, want to have more discussion about the material.
- Inside your organisation, consider 'work in progress' meetings and workshops. These are useful for disseminating your material and for collecting views within your own organisation. Alternatively, hold a launch event and invite a local celebrity to introduce your package.

Disseminating your resource at a national level can be more challenging. The costs can be high, and once you publicise the existence of the package you may have a lot of enquiries from patients and professionals outside your area. Consider what it will cost to send out the package. Will you need to charge people for it? If so, who will deal with distribution and with administering the payments?

The case study opposite demonstrates both the need to factor dissemination costs into your initial budget, and the downside to too much success.

Case study: Dissemination

Once the Nottingham children's bedwetting CD Rom was completed, it received a lot of publicity in the press and on radio. This publicity resulted in many public and professional requests for copies of the CD Rom and booklet. The development grant did not include money for dissemination and the developers found themselves with a successful product that they were unable to produce in sufficient numbers to satisfy demand.

Resource sharing

One of the keys to successful dissemination and publicity is to use already established distribution channels and communications networks. Going to one central organisation and persuading, or paying, them to assist is far easier than approaching individuals.

For example, if you wish to distribute your materials through pharmacies, approach your local pharmacy and find out about how they already receive resources. Some will come through their wholesalers, some through the Pharmacy Healthcare Scheme, others from pharmaceutical representatives. Don't be scared to think outside the box.

The following are some ways you can reach other people interested in the same topic if you decide that you want your material to have a wider audience.

National publicity

- Contact the **Centre for Health Information Quality** (CHIQ, *see* p 88) to find out about how to promote your resource at national level.
- Contact national patient and professional groups (*see* Useful contacts, p 103).
- Use the internet. Many patient information sites are now available on the internet. Speak to your IT developers about putting the information on your organisation's website or about identifying an appropriate service provider or space on the web if you don't have a website. This could result in a lot of attention – be sure that you want it! Also think about posting a message to some of the email discussion fora listed on p 24.

@
www.hpe.org.uk/calendar.
htm
www.hebs.org.uk/services/
events/index.htm

- Link your package to national awareness events. A diary of national events such as No Smoking Day or World Mental Health Day is available from Health Promotion Agencies.
- Enter for an award. Patient information packages may be eligible for the increasing number of awards listed below. Remember to look outside the normal range of health care awards, such as IT awards (*see* Multimedia, p 73). Although there is satisfaction and pleasure in it, submitting your package for an award can be time-consuming and expensive – especially if you have to travel to collect your prize!
- Take part in conferences and events on patient information. Increasingly, conferences are being organised on the topic of patient information itself or patient involvement developments. Depending on the medium you have chosen, you may consider conferences on video and multimedia.
- If you have the funding, or the connections, consider approaching a celebrity to promote your work. Think about personalities who (or whose families) have a particular personal interest in your area. But remember that if such information is in the public domain, they may be approached many times with similar requests. Respect their privacy. Also note than any negative publicity about them may reflect on your product. Alternatively, you could contact a media medic or the like (*see* A word of caution, p 54).

Case study: Using already established networks

To meet the demand for its bedwetting CD Rom, Nottingham paired up with ERIC – the Enuresis Resource and Information Centre. ERIC used its national and local networks to handle public and professional enquiries and to distribute copies of the CD Rom where appropriate.

Local publicity

- Contact local media. Prepare a press release about the package and send it to local newspapers and local radio stations. These media are especially interested in running personal interest stories. Keep a press file to reference appropriate articles. Local TV and radio are also useful for reaching distant audiences and minority ethnic groups. Asian radio stations, for example, are good ways of reaching these local communities.
- Arrange meetings with local groups. Offer to bring the package to meetings of groups such as PALS, voluntary health organisations and self-help groups.
- Consider approaching local NHS trusts, GP practices and pharmacies. NHS Walk-In and Health Living Centres may also promote your materials.
- Make the most of local meetings of medical and nursing staff. Make a presentation at any meetings of professional staff related to the clinical topic.

Further reading

Dixon-Woods M (1998). 'Dissemination of printed information for patients: a qualitative study of general practices'. *Health Education Journal*, vol 57, pp 16–30.

If you wish additional input to your communications strategy, try:

- **The Association of Healthcare Communicators (AHC)** – the primary independent network for healthcare communications professionals working in, or mainly with or for the NHS
- **The Institute of Public Relations**, for contact outside the NHS
- **The Newspaper Society**, which represents and promotes the interests of more than 1,300 regional and local, daily and weekly, paid-for and free titles.

See Useful contacts, p 103.

Awards

As mentioned above, a number of organisations now offer awards in the area of patient information. They include:

- **BMA Patient Information Award** – annual prize for the best patient information leaflets and booklets. The judging criteria are similar to those used by DISCERN (*see* p 85) but also look at presentation issues
- **BUPA Communications Award** – annual award for an achievement initiated and carried out by doctors associated with one or more of the Royal Colleges. Often such initiatives include the development of patient information
- **The Apple Patient Information Award** – set up by the Institute of Medical Illustrators in 2002 to recognise and reward medical illustrators who are required to produce interesting and effective patient information within the health care setting

- **Getting the Message Across** – this award, from the National Information Forum, calls attention to the information needs of disabled people and recognises initiatives that seek to bridge this gap
- **Plain English Campaign Awards** – for documents written in plain English that have not previously been awarded a Plain English Campaign Crystal Mark.
- **Medical Futures** recognises innovation in about ten healthcare categories. If you have a novel way of delivering patient information this may just be for you. In 2002, Sweet Talk (*see* Mobile health information, p 80) won two of the categories.
- **MediMedia's International Health and Medical Media Awards** – these are open to health and medical videos, films, CD Roms, or websites from around the world that address health or medical issues for consumers and health care professionals.

For contact details, *see* Useful contacts, p 103.

www.thefreddies.com

For details of awards for health information in other media and on the internet, *see* Multimedia (p 73) and The internet (p 77).

9 Evaluating and updating

People do not buy food that is past its sell by date, so why should they accept information that is not current? It is just as dangerous – if not more so. This section considers when and how to review your information on a regular basis and takes a brief tour of the ways you may want to more formally evaluate your product once it has been developed and distributed.

Annual review

Changes in the available research evidence and knowledge at local and/or national level make it essential to review your material regularly. This is especially true if a major new fact or treatment is identified, or an old one discounted. Once it has started to be used by patients, all patient information should ideally be reviewed after one year, and certainly after two years. The best way to ensure regular reviewing is to build it into an audit process or, as alluded to above, put an actual 'sell by' or 'review by' date on it.

The process of review involves a number of stages:

- **Stage one** – go back to the original aim for producing the information to assess whether it is being achieved, and whether or not it is meeting current needs. This will involve talking to patients using one of the methods described in Section 4.
- **Stage two** – check whether the material is being given to patients correctly. This will involve talking to health care professionals and observing how they give the information to patients.
- **Stage three** – check whether it is still up to date. This will involve a search for any clinical evidence that has changed since the package was produced and checking both local and national clinical guidelines on the topic of the information (*see* Section 4).
- **Stage four** – if regular reviews have not been included in organisational audits or reviews so far, try to make sure that patient information is included in future.

If you did not originally include a form in each copy of the resource to invite feedback, think about including one at the review stage. The case study opposite provides an excellent example of a feedback form and shows how the responses received provided improvements for subsequent editions.

Case study: Audience feedback

The booklet *You and Your Blood Pressure* was published by the Blood Pressure Association (BPA) when it launched in October 2000. The organisation printed 20,000 booklets and distributed them to health care professionals and consumers. A feedback form (*see* below) was included in the booklet and encouraged users to tell the BPA what they liked and disliked about the resource. About 4 per cent of consumers who received it provided the following insights into the booklet:

- It never clearly said exactly what the readings were for normal and high blood pressure. On re-reading it, the BPA realised that the patients were right, and they rectified this in their next print run.
- It was unrealistic about the side-effects of medications – either it was telling people too much, or it was not acknowledging that side-effects can be serious and make some people's lives miserable.
- People generally wanted more detail on various areas. It was not clear to readers that the booklet was meant to be general, and that other information that the BPA produced covered particular areas in more depth.
- There were lots of suggestions for additional places to distribute the booklet, such as their GP surgeries, nurse, pharmacies and other outlets.
- Some readers complained about the glossy paper as it was hard to write on it and it was difficult for people with poor eyesight because the light shone on it. Also it had some white text on a dark background and again this was difficult for people with visual problems.

15 SAMPLE FEEDBACK FORM

FEEDBACK FORM

We would like to know what you thought of this booklet. Any comments that you have will help us to make sure we are providing you with the right information, written in the right way.

Please fill in the form below, by ticking the boxes, and return to the **Blood Pressure Association** at the address given. **Thank you**

Where did you get this booklet from?

☐ GP   ☐ Practice nurse   ☐ Surgery waiting room

☐ Hospital consultant or nurse   ☐ Directly from the Blood Pressure Association

☐ Other

Was the information in this booklet:

☐ Too simple?   ☐ Just right?   ☐ Too difficult to understand?

Was the tone, or the 'voice', of the booklet:

☐ Not serious enough?   ☐ Just right?   ☐ Too serious?

Did the illustrations and tables, and the way that the information was set out, make it easy to understand?

☐ Yes   ☐ No   ☐ Not sure

Did the booklet answer the questions that you had about blood pressure?

☐ Yes   ☐ No   ☐ Not sure

If you answered **no** to the question above, what areas were not covered in the booklet?

(Please tear here)

FEEDBACK FORM CONTINUED

If you had a family member or friend with high blood pressure, would you suggest that they read this booklet?

☐ Yes   ☐ No   ☐ Not sure

When you finished reading this booklet, how much more did you feel that you understood about your high blood pressure?

☐ A lot more?   ☐ A little bit more?   ☐ About the same?   ☐ Less?

Which of the following services would you use if you wanted further information about high blood pressure?

☐ Telephone helpline   ☐ Group meetings ☐ Website

☐ Audio tape/video   ☐ Information in a foreign language

If you have ticked the box for information in a foreign language, which language?

Thank you for taking the time to fill this out.

If you have any further comments to make about the booklet, please use the space below.

Return the form to: Blood Pressure Association, 60 Cranmer Terrace, Tooting, London SW17 0QS

Source: The Blood Pressure Association

Action points

- Plan the timing of the reviews.
- Check with patients that the information still meets their needs.
- Check that the evidence base has not changed.
- Check that the information is still being given to patients at the right time.
- Reassess how many copies of the material you will need each year, and how much they will cost to provide.

Further reading

Beenstock J *et al* (1998). *In the Clear*. Manchester: South Manchester University Hospitals Trust.

Entwistle VA, Sowden AJ, Watt IS (1998). 'Evaluating interventions to promote patient involvement in decision-making: by what criteria should effectiveness be judged?'. *Journal of Health Services Research and Policy*, vol 3, pp 100–7.

Evaluation methods

From the outset, you should build in evaluation of the material you produce. A brief overview of some of the terms, and methods commonly used to do this can be found below, but it is important to seek appropriate expertise if you have not done this before. Colleagues within your own organisation may have research experience. Alternatively, ask a local university department.

There are two main forms of evaluation: formative and summative. Mays *et al* (1997) distinguish between them thus:

- formative evaluation is usually built in to project development and is more concerned with process, for example, testing a draft to obtain feedback before finalising it
- summative evaluation is normally used to assess the outcome(s) of a project and is more concerned with determining the effects on or impact of a package or a project.

Formative evaluation

If you have followed this guide, you will have carried out some of the elements of formative evaluation by:

- continuously getting feedback on your draft material from patients and from the other people, such as advisers and team members who have been working with you.

Summative evaluation

This is usually carried out once the work has been completed and there are several ways in which you can do it (*see* Section 4). However, first you have to determine what you want to measure.

What to measure

There is a range of outcome measures for evaluating patient information. As explained in Section 4, it is better to use previously validated questionnaires than to devise your own.

Things you could measure in patients include changes in:

- satisfaction, both overall and specifically with the resources themselves
- knowledge
- degree of decision-making
- degree of involvement
- clinical outcomes, such as anxiety or pain levels.

Differences in the type of information package you have developed, and where it is obtained, will also determine what measures to use. For example, measures about resources on surgery could be applied pre- and post-operatively, and two weeks after discharge. Materials informing people with asthma on their inhaler technique could be tested when given initially and then again six months later, to see if the information is still retained.

Also invite comments from health care professionals about ways in which they may have used the information, whether it has altered their practice in any way and whether they have found it useful.

Another reason for asking for additional help is to ensure that the questions you decide to ask – and indeed, the way in which you ask them – remain as unbiased as possible. Polit and Hugler (1998) suggest that all researchers are biased in relation to their own studies because of their intense interest in their research topics. As the following extract illustrates, it is easy to lose objectivity when so closely involved in a project.

> *Patient involvement is an emotive topic and the possibility that measures of effect will be selected in order to prove its advantage or disadvantage cannot be ignored. Evaluations of interventions should reflect, but not be unduly constrained by, their intended purposes and the frameworks within which their likely effects are viewed... Attempts should be made to ascertain which potential effects patients and health care professionals consider most important.*

Entwistle, Sowden and Watt (1998)

How to measure

To evaluate your patient information, use one of the methods outlined in Section 4. You might also consider using routinely collected statistics to evaluate the impact of your material – for instance, the number of visits people have made to outpatient clinics, or the number of prescriptions for drugs treating their conditions. Dunning *et al* (1999) give a more detailed description of the ways of carrying out this kind of evaluation.

The most thorough evaluation of the outcomes of any clinical intervention is the randomised controlled trial (RCT). Such trials involve the random allocation of patients to one group that receives the new intervention, and another that does not. Often neither patients nor doctors know which group is which during the trial. Although such evaluations are the most rigorous if they are conducted properly, they take two or three years to carry out and are expensive. Most producers of patient information will not be able to afford to evaluate their material in this way. Without an RCT you will not be able to reliably assess whether or not patients' behaviour has changed as a result of the information you have developed. However, this does not mean that you cannot evaluate other outcomes for patients using your information.

As well as evaluating the content of the package, you might wish to evaluate the process of development. For example, how much did the project cost and how well did the team work? You may wish to invite an independent evaluator to do this because their assessment will not be coloured by the experience of the development.

Action points

- Build formative evaluation into your project design at the start.
- Be clear about what you want to achieve with your evaluation so you can collect the appropriate data.
- Think through the most appropriate questions and design for a summative evaluation to be used at the end of the development, using one or more of the methods discussed on the previous page and in Section 4.

HEBS Research and Evaluation Toolbox – produced by the Health Education Board for Scotland (HEBS) to help practitioners in health and related fields think through how research can help them in planning and evaluating their work @ www.hebs.scot.nhs.uk/retoolbox/index.cfm

Further reading

There have been many research studies evaluating patient resources. Some examples of recent UK studies:

Burton AK, Waddell G, Tillotson KM, Summerton N (1999). 'Information and advice to patients with back pain can have a positive effect. A randomized controlled trial of a novel educational booklet in primary care'. *Spine*, vol 24, pp 2484–91.

Gillies MA, Baldwin FJ (2001). 'Do patient information booklets increase perioperative anxiety?' *European Journal of Anaesthesiology*, vol 18, pp 620–2.

Graham W, Smith P, Kamal A, Fitzmaurice A, Smith N, Hamilton N (2000). 'Randomised controlled trial comparing effectiveness of touch screen system with leaflet for providing women with information on prenatal tests'. *BMJ*, vol 320, pp 155–60.

Heaney D, Wyke S, Wilson P, Elton R, Rutledge P (2001). 'Assessment of impact of information booklets on use of healthcare services: randomised controlled trial'. *BMJ*, vol 322, pp 1218–21.

Hutchison C, Campbell S (2002). 'Evaluation of an information booklet for patients considering participation in phase I clinical trials in cancer'. *European Journal of Cancer Care (Engl.)* vol 11, pp 131–8.

Joshi HB, Newns N, Stainthorpe A, MacDonagh RP, Keeley FX Jr, Timoney AG (2001). 'The development and validation of a patient-information booklet on ureteric stents'. *British Journal of Urology International*, vol 88, pp 329–34.

Latthe M, Latthe PM, Charlton R (2000). 'Quality of information on emergency contraception on the Internet'. *British Journal of Family Planning*, vol 26, pp 39–43.

Martin J (2002). 'Randomized controlled trials: an introduction'. *Practice Nursing*, pp 401–7. This provides an excellent overview, and glossary of terms, for RCTs.

Nicholas D, Huntington P, Williams P, Vickery P (2001). 'Health information: an evaluation of the use of touch screen kiosks in two hospitals'. *Health Information Libraries Journal*, vol 18, pp 213–9.

Polit DF and Hugler BP (1998). *Nursing Research: Principles and methods*. Philadelphia: JB Lippincott.

Smart JM, Burling D (2001). 'Radiology and the internet: a systematic review of patient information resources'. *Clinical Radiology*, vol 56, pp 867–70.

Listings

→

Useful contacts

Aberdeen University
Health Services Research Unit
Medical School
Forester Hill
Aberdeen AB25 2ZD
Tel: 01224 681818
Email: hsru@abdn.ac.uk
Web: www.abdn.ac.uk/hsru

Age Concern England
Astral House
1268 London Road
London SW16 4ER
Tel: 0800 009966
Web: www.ageconcern.org.uk

Association of British Pharmaceutical
Industry (ABPI)
12 Whitehall
London SW1A 2DY
Tel: 020 7930 3477
Email: use query form on website
Web: www.abpi.org.uk

Association of Health Care Communicators
PO Box 265
Oxford OX1 5XB
Email: katherine.baldwin@virgin.net
Web: www.assochealth.org.uk

Association of Information Officers in the
Pharmaceutical Industry (AIOPI)
PO Box 297
Slough PDO SL1 7XT
Email: aiopi@aiopi.org.uk
Web: www.aiopi.org.uk

Audit Commission
1 Vincent Square
London SW1P 2PN
Tel: 020 7828 1212
Email: enquiries@audit-commission.gov.uk
Web: www.audit-commission.gov.uk

Australian National Health and Medical
Research Council (NHMRC)
Executive Secretary
Office of NHMRC (MDP 100)
GPO Box 9848
Canberra ACT 2601
Tel: +61 2 6289 9184
Email: exec.sec@nhmrc.gov.au

Bandolier (Evidence-based health care)
Pain Research
The Churchill
Oxford OX3 7LJ
Email: Bandolier@pru.ox.ac.uk
Web: www.jr2.ox.ac.uk/bandolier

Basic Skills Agency (BSA)
Commonwealth House
1–19 New Oxford Street
London WC1A 1NU
Tel: 020 7405 4017
Email: enquiries@basic-skills.co.uk
Web: www.basic-skills.co.uk

Books Beyond Words Series
The Royal College of Psychiatrists
17 Belgrave Square
London, SW1X 8PG
Tel: 020 7245 1231
Email: publications@rcpsych.ac.uk
Web: www.rcpsych.ac.uk/publications/bbw

British Association of Picture Libraries and
Agencies (BAPLA)
18 Vine Hill
London EC1R 5DZ
Tel: 020 7713 1780
Email: enquiries@bapla.org.uk
Web: www.bapla.org.uk

British Computer Society
1 Sanford Street
Swindon SN1 1HJ
Tel: 01793 417417
Email: bcshq@hq.bcs.org.uk
Web: www1.bcs.org.uk

British Copyright Council
29–33 Berners Street
London W1T 3AB
Tel: 01986 788122
Email: copyright@bcc2.demon.co.uk
Web: www.britishcopyright.org.uk

British Interactive Multimedia Association (BIMA)
Briarlea House
South Green
Billericay CM11 2PR
Email: info@bima.co.uk
Web: www.bima.co.uk

British Medical Association (BMA) Patient Information Award
BMA Library
BMA House
Tavistock Square
London WC1H 9JP
Tel: 020 7387 4499
Email: richard.jones@bma.org.uk
Web: www.bma.org.uk

BMJ Publishing Group
BMA House
Tavistock Square
London WC1H 9JP
Tel: 020 7383 6185 (enquiries)
    020 7383 6244 (bookshop)
    020 7383 6270 (subscriptions)
Web: www.bmjpg.com

BodyOnline
5 Moorside Court
Somerset Road
London W13 9PJ
Tel: 020 8567 8691
Web: www.bodyonline.co.uk

Bromley Health Management
17 South Street
Bromley
Kent BR1 1RH
Tel: 0800 9803447
Email: mailto:info@betterhealth.ltd.uk
Web: www.betterhealth.ltd.uk/bromley.htm

BUPA Foundation
BUPA House
15–19 Bloomsbury Way
London WC1A 2BA
Tel: 020 7656 2591
Email: saunderl@bupa.com
Web: www.bupafoundation.com

Cancer BACUP
3 Bath Place
Rivington Street
London EC2A 3DR
Tel: 020 7696 9003
Email: use form on website
Web: www.bacup.org.uk

Carers UK
20–25 Glasshouse Yard
London EC1A 4JT
Tel: 020 7490 8818
Email: info@ukcarers.org
Web: www.carersonline.org.uk

Central Office of Research Ethics Committees (COREC)
Room 76, B Block
40 Eastbourne Terrace
London W2 3QR
Tel: 020 7725 3431
Email: queries@corec.org.uk
Web: www.corec.org.uk/index.htm

Centre for Evidence Based Dermatology
BADPIG Project Co-ordinator
Ward C51, South Block
Queen's Medical Centre
Nottingham NG7 2UH
Tel: 0115 924 9924
Email: pippa.hemingway@nottingham.ac.uk
Web: www.nottingham.ac.uk/dermatology

Centre for Health Information Quality (CHIQ)
The Help for Health Trust
Highcroft
Romsey Road
Winchester
Hampshire SO22 5DH
Tel: 01962 863 511 x200
Email: chiq@chfht.org.uk
Web: www.hfht.org/chiq

Centre for Reviews and Dissemination (CRD)
University of York
York YO1 5DD
Tel: 01904 433634
Email: revdis@york.ac.uk
Web: www.york.ac.uk/inst/crd

Change
Block D
Hatcham Park Mews
London SW14 5QA
Tel: 020 7639 4312
Email: londonoffice@changepeople.co.uk
Web: www.changepeople.co.uk

**Chartered Society of Physiotherapy
Research and Clinical Effectiveness Unit**
14 Bedford Row
London WC1R 4ED
Tel: 020 7306 6155
Email: lis@csp.org.uk
Web: www.csp.org.uk

Cochrane Collaboration
The UK Cochrane Centre
Summertown Pavilion
Middle Way
Oxford OX2 7LG
Tel: 01865 516 300
Email: general@cochrane.co.uk

Cochrane Collaboration Consumer Network
PO Box 96
Burwood VIC 3125
Australia
Tel: +61 (0) 3 9885 5588
Email: info@cochraneconsumer.com

College of Health
St Margaret House
21 Old Ford
London E2 9PL
Tel: 020 8983 1225
Web: www.collegeofhealth.org.uk

Colon Cancer Concern
9 Rickett Street
London SW6 1RU
Tel: 020 7381 9711
Email: queries@coloncancer.org.uk
Web: www.coloncancer.org.uk

Commission for Health Improvement
1st Floor, Finsbury Tower
103–105 Bunhill Row
London, EC1Y 8TG
Tel: 020 7448 9200
Email: information@chi.nhs.uk
Web: www.chi.nhs.uk

Commission for Racial Equality
St Dunstan's House
201–211 Borough High Street
London SE1 1GZ
Tel: 020 7939 0000
Email: info@cre.gov.uk
Web: www.cre.gov.uk

**Communication Research Institute of
Australia (London)**
Tel: 07734 171854
Email: k.loglisci@communication.org.au

Consumation
53 Hosack Road
London SW17 7QW
Tel: 020 8673 4403
Email: david.dickinson@consumation.com

**Consumer Health Information Consortium
(CHIC)**
CHIC Treasurer
c/o Lambeth, Southwark and Lewisham
Health Authority
1 Lower Marsh
London SE1 7NT
Tel: 020 7928 9292 x 2507
Web: http://omni.ac.uk/CHIC/

Consumers for Ethics in Research (CERES)
PO Box 1365
London N16 0BW
Email: info@ceres.org.uk
Web: www.ceres.org.uk

Contact a Family (CaF)
209–211 City Road
London EC1V 1JN
Tel: 020 7608 8700
      0808 808 3555 (helpline)
Email: info@cafamily.org.uk
Web: www.cafamily.org.uk

Council for Disabled Children (CDC)
c/o National Children's Bureau
8 Wakeley Street
London EC1V 7QE
Tel: 020 7843 1900
Email: cdc@ncb.org.uk
Web: www.ncb.org.uk/cdc

Critical Appraisal Skills Programme (CASP)
Public Health Resource Unit
Institute of Health Sciences
Headington
Oxford OX3 7LF
Tel: 01865 226 968
Email: learning@phru.anglox.nhs.uk
Web: www.phru.org.uk/learning

CTIC Medicine
(Computers in Teaching Initiative)
Institute for Learning and Research
Technology
University of Bristol
8 Woodland Road
Bristol BS8 1TN
Tel: 0117 928 7492
Email: cticm@bristol.ac.uk

Datamonitor
Charles House
108–110 Finchley Road
London NW3 5JJ
Tel: 020 7675 7000
Email: eurinfo@datamonitor.com
Web: www.datamonitor.com

Designers in Health
Tel: 0151 707 1555 ext 116
      0114 271 3919
Email: andrew.dineley@btinternet.com
         brian.parkinson@sth.nhs.uk
Web: www.dihnet.org.uk

DIPEx
Department of Primary Care
Institute of Health Sciences
University of Oxford
Headington
Oxford OX3 7LF
Tel: 01865 226672
Email: dipex@dphpc.ox.ac.uk
Web: www.dipex.org

Directory of Social Change
24 Stephenson Way
London NW1 2DP
Tel: 020 7391 4900
Web: www.dsc.org.uk

Disability Rights Commission
DRC Helpline
Freepost MID 02164
Stratford-upon-Avon CV37 9HY
Tel: 08457 622633
Textphone: 08457 622644
Email: enquiry@drc-gb.org
Web: www.drc-gb.org

Doctor Patient Partnership
Tavistock House
Tavistock Square
London WC1 9TP
Tel: 020 7383 6803/6144
Email: dpp@bma.org.uk
Web: www.dpp.org.uk

Dr Foster Ltd
Sir John Lyon House
5 High Timber Street
London EC4V 3NX
Tel: 020 7557 4750
Email: info@drfoster.co.uk
Web: www.drfoster.co.uk

Dumas Ltd
Patman House
23–27 Electric Parade
George Lane
London E18 2LS
Tel: 020 8530 7589
Email: info@dumasltd.com
Web: www.dumasltd.com

Eden Communications
1 Harley Street
London W1N 1DA
Email: info@eden-communications.com
Web: www.eden-communications.com

Eido Healthcare Limited
19–21 Main Street
Keyworth
Nottinghamshire NG12 5AA
Tel: 0115 878 9052
Web: www.eidohealthcare.com

EITI Ltd
EITI House
Bridgegate
Howden
East Yorkshire DN14 7AE
Tel: 0870 701 2020
Email: hello@talkbackuk.info
Web: www.eiti.com

Elfrida Society, The
The Tom Blythe Centre
34 Islington Park Street
London N1 1PX
Tel: 020 7359 7443
Email: elfrida@elfrida.com
Web: www.elfrida.com

Enuresis Resource and Information Centre (ERIC)
34 Old School House
Britannia Road
Kingswood
Bristol
BS15 8DB
Tel: 0117 960 3060 (helpline)
Email: info@eric.org.uk
Web: www.eric.org.uk

Equal Opportunities Commission
Arndale House
Arndale Centre
Manchester M4 3EQ
Tel: 0845 601 5901
Email: info@eoc.org.uk
Web: www.eoc.org.uk

EQUIP (Electronic Quality Information for Patients)
Intelligence Officer for Patient Information
Regional Library Unit
Public Health Building
University of Birmingham
Birmingham B15 2TT
Tel: 0121 414 7754
Web: www.equip.nhs.uk

Factor V
XXV House
25 Langdale Gardens
Hove BN3 4HJ
Tel: 01237 236 624
Web: www.factorv.co.uk

Family Planning Association (FPA)
2–12 Pentonville Road
London N1 9FP
Tel: 020 7837 5432
Web: www.fpa.org.uk

Fife Primary Care NHS Trust
Health Promotion Department
Haig House
Cameron Bridge
Leven
Fife KY8 5RA
Tel: 01592 712812
Web: www.fife-hpd.demon.co.uk

Focus TV (FTV Ltd)
Old Garden Court
St Albans
Hertfordshire AL1 3HY
Tel: 01727 810101
Email: info@ftv.co.uk
Web: www.focus-tv.co.uk

Foundation for Informed Medical Decision Making
Health Dialog
60 State Street
11th Floor, Suite 700
Boston, MA 02109
Tel: +1 617 854 7440
Email: weborder@healthdialog.com
Web: www.healthdialog.com

GP & Specialist Info Limited
31 East Parade
Harrogate HG1 5LQ
Tel: 01423 562003
Email: info@specialistinfo.com
Web: www.specialistinfo.com

Health Action International – Europe (HAI)
Jacob van Lennepkade 334-T
1053 NJ Amsterdam
The Netherlands
Tel: + 31 20 683 3684
Email: info@haiweb.org
Web: www.haiweb.org

Health Coalition Initiative (HCI)
28 Queensbury Street
London N1 3AD
Tel: 020 7688 9208
Email: tinafunnell@cs.com

Health Development Agency
Holborn Gate
330 High Holborn
London WC1V 7BA
Tel: 020 7430 0850
Email: communications@hda-online.org.uk
Web: www.hda-online.org.uk

Health Education Board for Scotland (HEBS)
Woodburn House
Canaan Lane
Edinburgh EH10 4SG
Tel: 0131 536 5500
Email: infoservices@hebs.scot.nhs.uk
Web: www.hebs.scot.nhs.uk

Health Promotion Agency for Northern Ireland
18 Ormeau Avenue
Belfast BT2 8HS
Tel: 028 9031 1611
Email: info@hpani.org.uk
Web: www.healthpromotionagency.org.uk

Health Promotion in Wales
National Assembly for Wales
Cathays Park
Cardiff CF10 3NQ
Tel: 029 2068 1245
Email: hplibrary@wales.gsi.gov.uk
Web: www.hpw.wales.gov.uk

Health Quality Service (HQS)
15 Whitehall
London SW1A 2DD
Tel: 020 7389 1000
Web: www.hqs.org.uk

Healthwise
85–89 Duke Street
Liverpool L1 5AP
Tel: 0151 703 7777
Email: info@healthwise.org.uk
Web: www.healthwise.org.uk

Help for Health Trust
Highcroft
Romsey Road
Winchester
Hampshire SO22 5DH
Tel: 01962 849 100
Email: admin@hfht.org
Web: www.hfht.org

Help the Aged
207–221 Pentonville Road
London N1 9UZ
Tel: 020 7278 1114
Email: info@helptheaged.org.uk
Web: www.helptheaged.org.uk

Information Commissioner
Wycliffe House
Water Lane
Wilmslow
Cheshire SK9 5AF
Tel: 01625 545 700
      01625 545 745 (information)
Email: data@dataprotection.gov.uk
Web: www.dataprotection.gov.uk

Institute of Medical Illustrators
Email: enquiries@imi.org.uk
Web: www.imi.org.uk

Institute of Medicine, Law and Bio-ethics (IMLAB)
IMLAB Administrator
Liverpool Law School
University of Liverpool
Liverpool L69 7ZS
Tel: 0151 794 2302
Email: manny@liverpool.ac.uk
Web: www.liv.ac.uk/law/units/imlab.htm

Institute of Public Relations
The Old Trading House
15 Northburgh Street
London EC1V 0PR
Tel: 020 7253 5151
Email: info@ipr.org.uk
Web: www.ipr.org.uk

Institute of Translation and Interpreting
Fortuna House
South Fifth Street
Milton Keynes
England MK9 2EU
Tel: 01908 325250
Email: info@iti.org.uk
Web: www.iti.org.uk

INTRAN (Interpretation and Translation Agency for Public Services of Norfolk)
4 Heigham Street
Capital House
Unit 14
Norwich NR2 4TE
Tel: 01603 767477
Email: intran@norfolk.gov.uk

Irish Patients' Association
22–24 Lower Mount Street
Dublin 2
Ireland
Tel: + 353 (0)1661 0662
Email: stephenmcmahon@eircom.net
Web:www.stjames.ie/PatientServices/
    IrishPatientsAssociation

King's Fund Library
11–13 Cavendish Square
London W1M 0AN
Tel: 020 7307 2400
Email: libenq1@kehf.org.uk
Web: www.kingsfund.org.uk

Language Line Limited
Swallow House
11–21 Northdown Street
London N1 9BN
Tel: 020 7520 1430
Email: info@languageline.co.uk
Web: www.languageline.co.uk

Leicester University
University Road
Leicester LE1 7RH
Tel: 0116 252 2522
Web: www.le.ac.uk

Library Association of Ireland
53 Upper Mount Street
Dublin 2
Ireland
Tel: + 353 (0)86 607 0462
Web: www.libraryassociation.ie

Long-Term Medical Conditions Alliance (LMCA)
Unit 212
16 Baldwins Gardens
London EC1N 7RJ
Tel: 020 7813 3637
Email: info@lmca.org.uk
Web: www.lmca.org.uk

Macmillan Cancer Relief
89 Albert Embankment
London SE1 7UQ
Tel: 020 7840 7840
Email: cancerline@macmillan.org.uk
Web: www.macmillan.org.uk

Makaton Vocabulary Development Project (MVDP)
31 Firwood Drive
Camberley
Surrey GU15 3Q
Tel: 01276 61390
Email: mvdp@makaton.org
Web: www.makaton.org

Medical Defence Union (MDU)
230 Blackfriars Road
London SE1 8PJ
Tel: 020 7202 1500
Email: mdu@the-mdu.com
Web: www.the-mdu.com

Medical Futures
Email: mail@medicalfutures.co.uk
Web: www.medicalfutures.co.uk

Medical Research Council (MRC)
20 Park Crescent
London W1B 1AL
Tel: 020 7636 5422
Email: firstname.surname@headoffice.
    mrc.ac.uk
Web: www.mrc.ac.uk

Medicines Partnership
5th Floor
Royal Pharmaceutical Society
1 Lambeth High Street
London SE1 7JN
Tel: 020 7572 2474
Email: info@medicines-partnership.org
Web: www.medicines-partnership.org

Mediscan
Medical-On-Line Ltd
2nd Floor, Patman House
23–27 Electric Parade
George Lane
London E18 2LS
Tel: 020 8530 7589
Email: info@mediscan.co.uk
Web: www.mediscan.co.uk

Mental Health Foundation
7th Floor
83 Victoria Street
London SW1H 0HW
Tel: 020 7802 0300
Email: mhf@mhf.org.uk
Web: www.mentalhealth.org.uk

MIND
15–19 Broadway
London E15 4BQ
Tel: 020 8519 2122
Email: contact@mind.org.uk
Web: www.mind.org.uk

NAM Publications
16a Clapham Common Southside
London SW4 7AB
Tel: 020 7627 3200
Email: info@nam.org.uk
Web: www.aidsmap.com

National Association of Patient Participation (NAPP)
PO Box 999
Nuneaton CV11 5ZD
Tel: 01628 522663
Email: roger.battye@napp.org.uk
Web: www.napp.org.uk

National Asthma Campaign (NAC)
Providence House
Providence Place
London N1 0NT
Tel: 020 7226 2260
      0131 226 2544 (NAC Scotland)
Web: www.asthma.org.uk

National Cancer Alliance
PO Box 579
Oxford OX4 1LB
Tel: 01865 793 566
Email: nationalcanceralliance
      @btinternet.com
Web: www.nationalcanceralliance.co.uk

National Consumer Council
20 Grosvenor Gardens
London SW1
Tel: 020 7730 3469
Email: info@ncc.org.uk
Web: www.ncc.org.uk

National Institute for Clinical Excellence (NICE)
11 Strand
London WC2N
Tel: 020 7766 9191
Email: nice@nice.nhs.uk
Web: www.nice.org.uk

National Patient Safety Agency (NPSA)
Marble Arch Tower
55 Bryanston Street
London W1H 7AJ
Tel: 020 7868 2203
Email: enquires@npsa.org.uk
Web: www.npsa.org.uk

Newspaper Society
Bloomsbury House
74–77 Great Russell Street
London WC1B 3DA
Tel: 020 7636 7014
Email: ns@newspapersoc.org.uk
Web: www.newspapersoc.org.uk/index.html

NHS 24 (Scotland)
Tel: 0845 424242
Web: www.nhs24.com

NHS Direct
Tel: 0845 4647
Web: www.nhsdirect.nhs.uk

NHS Executive Headquarters
Quality and Consumers Branch
Quarry House
Quarry Hill
Leeds LS2 7UE
Tel: 0113 254 5000

NHS Information Authority (NHSIA)
Aqueous II
Aston Cross
Rocky Lane
Birmingham B6 5RQ
Tel: 0121 333 0333
Email: information@nhsia.nhs.uk
Web: www.nhsia.nhs.uk

NHS Regional Libraries Group
John Rylands University of Manchester
Oxford Road
Manchester M13 9PP
Tel: 0161 275 3717
Web: www.londonlinks.ac.uk/rlg/index.htm

National Information Forum
Post Point 10/10
BT Burne House
Bell Street
London NW1 5BZ
Tel: 020 7402 6681
Web: www.nif.org.uk

Norfolk County Council
Communications Unit
Chief Executive's Department
County Hall
Martineau Lane
Norwich NR1 2DH
Tel: 01603 222949
Email: information@norfolk.gov.uk
Web: www.norfolk.gov.uk

Patient Concern
PO Box 23732
London SW5 9FY
Tel: 020 7373 0794
Email: patientconcern@hotmail.com
Web: www.patientconcern.org.uk

Patient Information Forum (P*i*F)
Co-ordinator
28 Queensbury Street
London N1 3AD
Tel: 020 7688 9208
Email: tinafunnell@btopenworld.com
Web: www.soi.city.ac.uk/~mjl/pif.htm

Patient Information Publications (PIP)
25 Polwarth Crescent
Brunton Park
Newcastle upon Tyne NE3 2EE
Tel: 0191 217 1536
Email: patientuk@btinternet.com
Web: www.patient.co.uk

Patients' Association (PA)
PO Box 935
Harrow HA1 3YJ
Helpline tel: 020 8423 8999
Admin tel: 020 8423 9111
Email: mailbox@patients-association.com
Web: www.patients-association.com

Patients' Forum
Riverbank House
1 Putney Bridge Approach
London SW6 3JD
Tel: 020 7736 7903
Email: info@thepatientsforum.org.uk
Web: www.thepatientsforum.org.uk

People First
PO Box 5200
Northampton NN1 1ZB
Tel: 01604 721 666
Email: northants@peoplefirst.org.uk
Web: www.peoplefirst.org.uk

Pharmacy Healthcare Scheme
Royal Pharmaceutical Society of Great Britain
1 Lambeth High Street
London SE1 7JN
Tel: 020 7572 2265
Email: phs@rpsgb.org.uk

Plain English Campaign (PEC)
PO Box 3
New Mills
High Peak
Derbyshire SK22 4QP
Tel: 01663 744 409
Email: info@plainenglish.co.uk
Web: www.plainenglish.co.uk

Plain Facts
c/o Norah Fry Research Centre
3 Priory Road
Bristol BS8 1TX
Tel: 0117 923 8137
Minicom: 0117 928 8856
Web: www.bris.ac.uk/Depts/NorahFry

Promoting Excellence in Consumer Medicines Information (pecmi)
53 Hosack Road
London SW17 7QW
Tel: 020 8673 4403
Email: david.dickinson@consumation.com
Web: www.pecmi.org

Proprietary Association of Great Britain (PAGB)
Vernon House
Sicilian Avenue
London WC1A 2QH
Tel: 020 7242 8331
Web: www.pagb.co.uk

Research Council on Complementary Medicines (RCCM)
60 Great Ormond Street
London WC1N 3JF
Tel: 020 7833 8897
Email: info@rccm.org.uk
Web: www.rccm.org.uk

Royal College of Psychiatrists
17 Belgrave Square
London SW1X 8PG
Tel: 020 7235 2351
Email: rcpsych@rcpsych.ac.uk
Web: www.rcpsych.ac.uk

Royal College of Surgeons
35 Lincoln's Inn Fields
London WC2A 3PE
Tel: 020 7405 3474
Web: www.rcseng.ac.uk

Royal National Institute of the Blind (RNIB)
105 Judd Street
London WC1H 9NE
Tel: 020 7388 1266
Email: helpline@rnib.org.uk
Web: www.rnib.org.uk

Royal National Institute for Deaf People (RNID)
19–23 Featherstone Street
London EC1Y 8SL
Tel: 020 7296 8000
Textphone: 020 7296 8001
Email: informationline@rnid.org.uk
Web: www.rnid.org.uk

Royal Pharmaceutical Society of Great Britain (RPSGB)
1 Lambeth High Street
London SE1 7JN
Tel: 020 7735 9141
Email: enquiries@rpsgb.org.uk
Web: www.rpsgb.org.uk

ScHARR Information Resources
University of Sheffield
Regent Court
30 Regent Street
Sheffield S1 4DA
Tel: 0114 222 5454
Email: scharrlib@sheffield.ac.uk
Web: www.shef.ac.uk/~scharr

Scottish Association of Health Councils (SAHC)
24 Palmerston Place
Edinburgh EH12 5AL
Tel: 0131 220 4101
Email: sahc@sol.co.uk
Web: www.show.scot.nhs.uk/sahc

Scottish Intercollegiate Guidelines Network (SIGN)
9 Queen Street
Edinburgh EH2 1JQ
Tel: 0131 225 7324
Email: d.service@rcpe.ac.uk
Web: www.sign.ac.uk

Scriptographic Publications Ltd
Channing House
Butts Road
Alton
Hampshire GU34 1ND
Tel: 0800 028 5670
Email: sales@scriptographic.co.uk
Web: www.scriptographic.co.uk

Society of Health Education and Health Promotion Specialists (SHEPS)
64 Terregles Avenue
Pollokshields
Glasgow G41 4LX
Web: www.hj-web.co.uk/sheps

Society of Public Information Networks (SPIN)
PO Box 2306
Chippenham SN14 7WA
Tel: 01249 783 702
Email: info@spin.org.uk
Web: www.spin.org.uk

Telephone Helplines Association (THA)
3rd/4th Floor
9 Marshalsea Road
London SE1 1EP
Tel: 020 7089 6321
Email: info@helplines.org.uk
Web: www.helplines.org.uk

Tim Albert Training
Paper Mews Court
284 High Street
Dorking
Surrey RH4 1QT
Tel: 01306 877993
Email: tatraining@cs.com
Web: www.timalbert.co.uk

Videos for Patients
Linkward Productions Limited
Yew Tree Cottage
School Lane
Bentley
Farnham GU10 5JP
Tel: 01420 520100
Email: info@linkward.co.uk
Web: www.linkward.co.uk/vfp.html

UK Council for Health Informatics Professions (UKCHIP)
Tel: 07884 438 052
Email: ukchipadmin@nhsia.nhs.uk
Web: www.primis.nottingham.ac.uk/ukchip

Wellcome Trust
The Wellcome Building
183 Euston Road
London NW1 2BE, UK
Tel: 020 7611 8888
Email: contact@wellcome.ac.uk
Web: www.wellcome.ac.uk

Wellcome Trust Medical Photographic Library
210 Euston Road
London NW1 2BE
Tel: 020 7611 8348
Email: medphoto.info@wellcome.ac.uk
Web: http://medphoto.wellcome.ac.uk

Sources for project funding

If you cannot fund your patient information development from within your organisation's resources, there are a number of places you can go to ask for financial support. The organisations listed below are the ones we know about that might be able to help.

Many areas have a Council for Voluntary Service that will have details of local and national trusts, and will know how you can access various computer databases, such as Funderfinder, that can search for grant-making trusts relevant your area of interest. You can also look at some of the following internet sites:

- **Charities Direct** is a free web service featuring financial and contact information on the UK's top 10,000 charities @ www.caritasdata.co.uk
- **Charity Choice** is an encyclopaedia of charities on the internet @ www.charitychoice.co.uk
- **The Charity Commission** exists to give the public confidence in the integrity of charities in England and Wales. It provides advice and publications @ www.charity-commission. gov.uk
- **RDInfo** is funded by the Department of Health and provides researchers with direct access to up-to-the-minute information on health-related funding and training opportunities. RDInfo, 34 Hyde Terrace, The Leeds Teaching Hospitals NHS Trust, Leeds LS2 9LN. Tel: 0113 3926379 @ www.rdinfo.org.uk

You may also want to think about partnering with other organisations with similar goals that, perhaps through their charitable status, may have access to different funding sources.

Further reading

There are several useful publications that list grant-giving agencies with details of the kinds of projects they support and when to apply for money. They include:

Fitzherbert L, Wickens J, eds (2003). *The Top 300 Trusts: 2003–2004*. London: Directory of Social Change.

Forrester and Pilch (1998). *A Guide to Funding from Government Departments and Agencies*. London: Directory of Social Change.

Most university and reference libraries will have copies of these and other directories of grant-making trusts, including grants from European sources.

Organisation listing

Association of Medical Research Charities
61 Gray's Inn Road
London WC1X 8TL
Tel: 020 7269 8820
Email: info@amrc.org.uk
Web: www.amrc.org.uk

BUPA Foundation
BUPA House
15–19 Bloomsbury Way
London WC1A 2BA
Tel: 0800 001010
Web: www.bupafoundation.com/html/
    funding/index.html

Department of Health – S64 General Scheme
Grants Administration Unit
Room 609 Wellington House
133–155 Waterloo Road
London SE1 8UG
Tel: 020 7972 4109
Web: www.doh.gov.uk/sect64/grants.htm

The scheme is restricted to those voluntary
organisations working in health and social
care in England. Patient and public
involvement is one of its priority areas.

Foundation of Nursing Studies
32 Buckingham Palace Road
London SW1W 0RE
Tel: 020 7233 5750
Email: admin@fons.org
Web: www.fons.org

For projects that involve nurses working to
improve patient care.

Gatsby Charitable Foundation
Allington House (1st Floor)
150 Victoria Street
London SW1E 5AE
Tel: 020 7410 0330
Email: contact@gatsby.org.uk
Web: www.gatsby.org.uk

Joseph Rowntree Foundation
The Homestead
40 Water End
York
North Yorkshire YO30 6WP
Tel: 01904 629241
Email: info@jrf.org.uk
Web: www.jrf.org.uk/funding

King's Fund Grants Department
11–13 Cavendish Square
London W1M 0AN
Tel: 020 7307 2495
Email: ZKhan@kingsfund.org.uk
Web: www.kingsfund.org.uk/eGrants/
    html/index.html

National Endowment for Science Technology and the Arts (NESTA)
Fishmongers' Chambers
110 Upper Thames Street
London EC4R 3TW
Tel: 020 7645 9538
Email: nesta@nesta.org.uk
Web: www.nesta.org.uk (go to 'Education')

National Lotteries Community Fund
St Vincent House
16 Suffolk Street
London SW1Y 4NL
Enquiries Line: 020 7747 5299
Minicom: 020 7747 5347
Email: enquiries@community-fund.org.uk
Web: www.community-fund.org.uk

New Opportunities Fund
1 Plough Place
London EC4A 1DE
Tel: 020 7211 1800
Email: general.enquiries@nof.org.uk
Web: www.nof.org.uk (go to 'Health')

NHS Research and Development Programme
Web: www.doh.gov.uk/research/index.htm

Details of current initiatives, funding
application procedures and other funders.

Nuffield Foundation
28 Bedford Square
London WC1B 3JS
Tel: 020 7631 0566
Web: www.nuffieldfoundation.org/grants

Nuffield Trust
59 New Cavendish Street
London W1G 7LP
Tel: 020 7631 8450
Email: mail@nuffieldtrust.org.uk
Web: www.nuffieldtrust.org.uk/
   grant_information/ grants.htm

PPP Foundation
13 Cavendish Square
London W1G OPQ
Tel: 020 7307 2622
Email: info@pppfoundation.org.uk
Web: www.pppfoundation.org.uk

Wellcome Trust
Grants Officer
The Wellcome Building
183 Euston Road
London NW1 2BE
Tel: 020 7611 8888
Email: contact@wellcome.ac.uk
Web: www.wellcome.ac.uk/en/1/gra.html

Useful websites

A vast array of health information is available on the internet. Relevant web addresses are given throughout the guide, but the following listing provides some additional starting points for those interested in this area. This list is by no means comprehensive; nor does it endorse those contained within it. Readers are also encouraged to look at Multimedia (p 73) for other sources of electronic information.

Web trends

Although web trends are constantly changing, a recent Datamonitor report (2002) indicates that at the time of publication a third of European and almost half of American consumers have used the internet to get health information in the past year. Consumers were reported to prefer sites such as the BBC and Yahoo to websites directly connected to pharmaceutical companies, government or medical institutions.

Useful sites

These sites have often been quoted as models of good practice and/or as useful sources of UK health information:

- **MS Society**: www.mssociety.org.uk
- **Teenage Health Freak**: www.teenagehealthfreak.org.uk
- **Well-aware**: www.well-aware.co.uk
- **Net Doctor**: www.netdoctor.co.uk
- **Medic Direct**: www.medicdirect.co.uk
- **Health Info 4 U**: www.healthinfo4u.org.uk

Government consumer health sites

- **NHS Direct Online** @ www.nhsdirect.nhs.uk, outlined in the Information for Health strategy (*see* p 10), is the UK Internet gateway to good quality information for the public. It allows access to NHS Direct services and forms the patient floor of the National Electronic Library for Health. Recently NHS Direct Online has started to offer an email enquiry service. Where appropriate, and where there is no value in replicating their work, NHSDO will point to the following websites from other English-speaking nations:
- **Health Insite** – the Australian Government's consumer health site, which splits information into different audience segments such as LifeStages, Population Groups, Lifestyle and Conditions @ www.healthinsite.gov.au
- **Healthfinder** – a free gateway to reliable health information developed by the US Department of Health & Human Services (DHHS). It links to carefully selected information from US government agencies, major non-profit organisations, state health departments and universities. It covers more than 1,000 topics and every link has been reviewed according to strict quality guidelines @ www.healthfinder.gov

- **MedlinePlus** – provided by the US National Library of Medicine, National Institutes for Health and the Department of Health and Human Services, this service provides a wide variety of health topics, drug information, dictionaries, directories and other resources, including information on clinical research studies @ www.medlineplus.com
- **The Canadian Health Network** – Canada Health's bilingual site which focuses on health promotion @ www.canadian-health-network.ca

Health promotion

- **The Society of Health Education and Health Promotion Specialists (SHEPS)** aims to advance good practice in health education and health promotion, including the development of good quality information @ www.hj-web.co.uk/sheps/index.html)
- **HealthPromis** is a national health promotion database for the UK, maintained by the Health Development Agency @ http://health)promis.hda-online.org.uk
- **The Health Education Board for Scotland** @ www.hebs.scot.nhs.uk/datasets
- **Health Promotion Agency for Northern Ireland** @ www.healthpromotionagency.org.uk/
- **Health Promotion Wales** @ www.hpw.wales.gov.uk

Patient information resources

- **The Wellcome Trust** offers some additional sources of information for health consumers on its databases @ www.wellcome.ac.uk/en/1/misinfrechecdbs.html
- **Scriptographic Publications** publish a range of booklets on health education and patient information issues @ www.scriptographic.co.uk
- **Dumas** are preparing 20 patient information leaflets in each of 22 specialties in digital formats @ www.dumasltd.com

Cancer

- **CancerBACUP patient information database** provides a guide to the books, booklets, factsheets, audio and videotapes that are available for cancer patients and their relatives in the UK @ www.cancerbacup.org.uk/resource/catalogue.htm
- **CHIQ and Macmillan** have also produced a directory that is intended primarily, but not exclusively, for use by health care professionals working in the field of cancer treatment and care, who have a role in providing information to people with cancer and those close to them @ www.hfht.org/macmillan/contents.htm

Dermatology

- **The British Association of Dermatologists Patient Information Gateway project (BADPIG)** – 'BADPIG' is the amusing acronym for a joint project between the Centre for Evidence Based Dermatology @ www.nottingham.ac.uk/dermatology and the British Association of Dermatology @ www.bad.org.uk whose aim is to produce the most easy to read, reliable and independent online source of information on skin diseases and their treatment.

Children

- **CaF Directory** is free on the internet, and updated monthly, including details of available support groups for more than 800 conditions affecting children. CaF also has local and national support networks @ www.cafamily.org.uk/dirworks.html
- **The Institute of Child Health and Great Ormond Street Hospital** provide an online factsheet service for a range of conditions, tests, operations and drugs @ www.ich.ucl.ac.uk/patients_fam/ppweb/html/fact_sheets.html#a
- **Online Information for Children – Great Ormond Street** @ www.goshkids.nhs.uk
- **Online Information for Children – Queens Medical Centre** @ www.chic-qmc.org.uk

Voluntary health organisations

- **NHS A–Z and Help-Direct** databases are available from the Help for Health Trust. 'Helpbox' is the standalone version @ www.hfht.org/databases
- **Patient Information Publications** provides details of self-help health organisations on the internet. A database of patient information leaflets (PILs) available to subscribers through software packages and on CD Rom @ www.mentor-update.com (Click on PILs)
- **UK Self Help Directory** lists 780 groups but sadly the site is undated @ www.ukselfhelp.info
- **Healthwise** is a directory of national health organisations, and those serving the north west, available to subscribers and updated monthly @ wwww.healthwise.org.uk

US consumer health databases

- **The consumer edition of Health Source**® claims to be the richest collection of consumer health information available to libraries worldwide. This priced resource provides access to nearly 200 full-text, consumer health periodicals primarily in the United States @ www.epnet.com/biomedical/hsconsumered.asp
- **The Health Reference Center** is a US product similar to Health Source®, above @ www.gale.com
- **The National Institutes of Health** provide a free and extensive consumer health information resource, also in the United States @ www.nih.gov/health/consumer

Television

For health sites in television, see:

- **BBC**: www.bbc.co.uk/health
- **Channel 4**: www.channel4.com/health
- **GMTV**: http://gm.tv
- **Discovery Health**: www.discoveryhealth.co.uk
- **Channel Health**: www.channelhealth.tv

Bibliography

This section lists those publications that are cited or referred to in the text and publications relating to the topic of patient information as a whole. For publications relating to specific areas within this topic, see Further reading selections at the relevant sections of the book.

More references relevant to this topic are listed below. There are many academic articles published; the emphasis in this book is on UK papers published in the last few years. Two additional resources for finding relevant information on this topic are PubMed and The British Medical Journal Online. Pubmed allows free searching of the Medline and PreMedline databases, giving brief details of articles. The British Medical Journal Online provides full text of its articles free of charge, including a searchable archive.

@ http://pubmed.gov

@ http://bmj.com/

Australian National Health and Medical Research Council (NHMRC) (2000). *How to Present the Evidence for Consumers: Preparation of consumer publications*. Canberra: NHMRC.

BBC/Macmillan Cancer Relief (1997). *The Cancer Guide*. London: BBC/Macmillan Cancer Relief.

Beenstock J (1998). *In the Clear*. Manchester: South Manchester University Hospitals Trust.

BMRB Qualitative for Macmillan Cancer Relief (March 1999). *Developing Information for The Cancer Guide*. London: Macmillan Cancer Relief.

Bragg J (1999). 'Preparing an information leaflet'. *Paediatric Nursing*, vol 11, pp 6–9.

Bryant LD, Murray J, Green JM, Hewison J, Sehmi I, Ellis A (2001). 'Descriptive information about Down syndrome: a content analysis of serum screening leaflets'. *Prenatal Diagnosis*, vol 21, pp 1057–63.

Bulmer PJ, James M, Ellis-Jones J, Smith D, Timoney AG, Donovan J (2001). 'A randomized trial comparing the effectiveness and preference of a touch-screen computer system with a leaflet for providing women with information on urinary symptoms suggestive of detrusor instability'. *BJU International*, vol 88, pp 532–5.

Callaghan P, Chan HC (2001). 'The effect of videotaped or written information on Chinese gastroscopy patients' clinical outcomes'. *Patient Education and Counseling*, vol 42, pp 225–30.

CHIQ (1999). *Topic Bulletin No 4*. Winchester: Centre for Health Information Quality.

Cooper H, Booth K, Fear S, Gill G (2001). 'Chronic disease patient education: lessons from meta-analyses'. *Patient Education and Counseling*, vol 44, 107–17.

Coulter A (1999). 'Paternalism or partnership?' *BMJ*, vol 319, pp 719–720.

Coulter A (2002). 'After Bristol: putting patients at the centre'. *BMJ*, vol 324, pp 648–51.

Coulter A, Entwistle V, Gilbert D (1998). *Informing Patients: An assessment of the quality of patient information materials*. London: King's Fund.

Datamonitor (2002). *The Internet and the Patient–Physician Relationship. Part 1: The patient's perspective*. Brief No. BFHC0487. New York: Datamonitor.

Davis JJ (2002). 'Disenfranchising the disabled: the inaccessibility of Internet-based health information'. *Journal of Health Communication*, vol 7, pp 355–67.

Delamothe T (2000). 'Quality of websites: kitemarking the west wind'. *BMJ*, vol 321, pp 843–4.

Department of Health (1999a) *Patient and Public Involvement in the New NHS*. London: The Stationery Office.

Department of Health (1999b) *Introducing Caldicott Guardians into the NHS*. Leeds: NHS Executive.

Department of Health (2001). *e-Business Strategy*. London: Department of Health.

Department of Health (2002a) *The NHS Plan. A plan for investment, a plan for reform*. London: The Stationery Office.

Department of Health (2002b) *Supporting the Implementation of Patient Advice and Liaison Services (PALS) – Core standards and practical guide*. London: The Stationery Office.

De Ruiter HP, Larsen KE (2002). 'Developing a transcultural patient care Web site'. *Journal of Transcultural Nursing*, vol 13, pp 61–7.

Dickinson D, Raynor DK, Duman M (2001). 'Patient information leaflets for medicines: using consumer testing to determine the most effective design'. *Patient Education and Counseling*, vol 43, pp 147–59.

Dixon-Woods M (2001). 'Writing wrongs? An analysis of published discourses about the use of patient information leaflets'. *Social Science and Medicine*, vol 52, pp 1417–32.

Dunning M, Abi-Aad G, Gilbert D, Hutton H, Brown C (1999). *Experience, Evidence and Everyday Practice*. London: King's Fund.

Eaton L (2002). 'NHS Direct Online explores partnerships with other health organisations'. *BMJ*, vol 324, p 568.

Eaton L (2002). 'UK government aims to integrate health information on the internet'. *BMJ*, vol 324, p 566.

Edwards A, Elwyn G, Mulley A (2002). 'Explaining risks: turning numerical data into meaningful pictures'. *BMJ*, vol 324, pp 827–30.

Entwistle VA, Sowden AJ, Watt IS (1998). 'Evaluating interventions to promote patient involvement in decision-making: by what criteria should effectiveness be judged?' *Journal of Health Services Research and Policy* vol 3 (2), pp 100–7.

Entwistle VA, Watt IS, Davis H, Dickson R, Pickard D, Rosser J (1998). 'Developing information materials to present the findings of technology assessments to consumers. The experience of the NHS Centre for Reviews and Dissemination'. *International Journal of Technology Assessment in Health Care*, vol 14, pp 47–70.

Fife Healthcare NHS Trust, Fife Health Board and the Health Education Board for Scotland (1995). *Getting Your Message Across*. Fife: Fife Healthcare NHS Trust, Fife Health Board and the Health Education Board for Scotland.

Fitzmaurice DA, Adams JL (2000). 'A systematic review of patient information leaflets for hypertension'. *Journal of Human Hypertension*, vol 14, pp 259–62.

Forster A, Smith J, Young J, Knapp P, House A, Wright J (2001). 'Information provision for stroke patients and their caregivers'. *Cochrane Database of Systematic Reviews*, vol 3, p CD001919.

Galimberti A, Jain S (2000). 'Gynaecology on the Net: evaluation of the information on hysterectomy contained in health-related web sites'. *Journal of Obstetrics and Gynaecology*, vol 20, pp 3–299.

Garrud P, Wood M, Stainsby L (2001). 'Impact of risk information in a patient education leaflet'. *Patient Education and Counseling*, vol 43, pp 301–4.

Harvey HD, Fleming P (2000). 'A rapid appraisal method for the selection and pre-testing of environmental health leaflets'. *Journal of the Royal Society for the Promotion of Health*, vol 120, pp 2–116.

Harvey HD, Fleming P, Cregan K, Latimer E (2000). 'The health promotion implications of the knowledge and attitude of employees in relation to health and safety leaflets'. *International Journal of Environmental Health Research*, vol 10, pp 4–329.

Hastings G, MacFadyen L (2002). 'Controversies in tobacco control: the limitations of fear messages'. *Tobacco Control*, vol 11, pp 73–5.

Hewison J, Cuckle H, Baillie C, Sehmi I, Lindow S, Jackson F, Batty J (2001). 'Use of videotapes for viewing at home to inform choice in Down syndrome screening: a randomised controlled trial'. *Prenatal Diagnosis*, vol 21, pp 146–9.

Hollins S (1996). *Going to the Doctor*. London: St George's Mental Health Library.

Hughes S (2002). 'The effects of giving patients pre-operative information'. *Nursing Standard*, vol 16(28), pp 33–7.

Humphris GM, Ireland FS, Field EA (2001a). 'Immediate knowledge increase from an oral cancer information leaflet in patients attending a primary health care facility: a randomised controlled trial'. *Oral Oncology*, vol 37, pp 99–102.

Humphris GM, Ireland FS, Field EA (2001b). 'Randomised trial of the psychological effect of information about oral cancer in primary care settings'. *Oral Oncology*, vol 37, pp 548–52.

Ives NJ, Troop M, Waters A, Davies S, Higgs C, Easterbrook PJ (2001). 'Does an HIV clinical trial information booklet improve patient knowledge and understanding of HIV clinical trials?' *HIV Medicine*, vol 2, pp 241–9.

Jaffray MA, Osman L, Mackenzie JF, Stearn R (2001). 'Asthma leaflets for patients: what do asthma nurses use?'. *Patient Education and Counseling*, vol 42, pp 193–8.

Jenkins JM (2002). 'ReproMED on the Internet today and tomorrow'. *Human Fertility*, vol 5, pp S66–S71.

Jones RB, Atkinson JM, Coia DA, Paterson L, Morton AR, McKenna K, Craig N, Morrison J, Gilmour WH (2001). 'Randomised trial of personalised computer based information for patients with schizophrenia'. *BMJ*, vol 322, pp 835–40.

Kalten MR, Ardito DA, Cimino C, Wylie-Rosett J (2000). 'A Web-accessible core weight management program'. *The Diabetes Educator*, vol 26, pp 929–36.

Kamel Boulos MN, Roudsari AV, Gordon C, Muir Gray JA (2001). 'The use of quality benchmarking in assessing web resources for the dermatology virtual branch library of the National electronic Library for Health (NeLH)'. *Journal of Medical Internet Research*, vol 3, E5.

Karp S, Monroe AF (2002). 'Quality of healthcare information on the Internet: caveat emptor still rules'. *Managed Care Quarterly*, vol 10, pp 3–8.

Krouse HJ (2001). 'Video modelling to educate patients'. *Journal of Advanced Nursing*, vol 33, pp 748–57.

Kruse AY, Kjaergard LL, Krogsgaard K, Gluud C, Mortensen EL, Gottschau A, Bjerg AM (2000). 'A randomized trial assessing the impact of written information on outpatients' knowledge about and attitude toward randomized clinical trials'. *Controlled Clinical Trials*, vol 21, pp 3–240.

Kunst H, Groot D, Latthe PM, Latthe M, Khan KS (2002). 'Accuracy of information on apparently credible websites: survey of five common health topics'. *BMJ*, vol 324, pp 581–2.

Lennox AS, Osman LM, Reiter E, Robertson R, Friend J, McCann I, Skatun D, Donnan PT (2001). 'Cost effectiveness of computer tailored and non-tailored smoking cessation letters in general practice: randomised controlled trial'. *BMJ*, vol 322, p 1396.

Little P, Roberts L, Blowers H, Garwood J, Cantrell T, Langridge J, Chapman J (2001). 'Should we give detailed advice and information booklets to patients with back pain? A randomized controlled factorial trial of a self-management booklet and doctor advice to take exercise for back pain'. *Spine*, vol 26, pp 2065–72.

Little P, Somerville J, Williamson I, Warner G, Moore M, Wiles R, George S, Smith A, Peveler R (2001). 'Randomised controlled trial of self management leaflets and booklets for minor illness provided by post'. *BMJ*, vol 322, pp 1214–7.

Llewellyn JS, Jones G, Donnelly P (2001). 'Questions patients ask psychiatrists'. *Psychiatric Bulletin*, vol 25, pp 1–24.

Macfarlane J, Holmes W, Gard P, Thornhill D, Macfarlane R, Hubbard R (2002). 'Reducing antibiotic use for acute bronchitis in primary care: blinded, randomised controlled trial of patient information leaflet'. *BMJ*, vol 324, pp 91–4.

Mackay D (2000). 'Consumer health information', in *Managing Knowledge in Health Services*, Andrew Booth, Graham Walton eds, pp 69–89. London: CILIP.

Mays N *et al* (1997). *Evaluating Primary Care Developments*. London: King's Fund.

McPherson A, Glazebrook C, Smyth A (2001). 'Double click for health: the role of multimedia in asthma education'. *Archives of Disease in Childhood*, vol 85, pp 447–9.

Newell R, Clarke M (2000). 'Evaluation of a self-help leaflet in treatment of social difficulties following facial disfigurement'. *International Journal of Nursing Studies*, vol 37, pp 381–8.

NHS (2002). *Toolkit for Producing Patient Information*. Available at: www.doh.gov.uk/nhsidentity

NHS Information Authority (2002) *Share with Care! People's views on consent and confidentiality of patient information*. Birmingham: NHS Information Authority.

North G, Magree G, Roe M (1996). 'Guidelines for producing patient information'. *Nursing Standard* vol 10 (47), pp 46–8.

O'Cathain A, Walters SJ, Nicholl JP, Thomas KJ, Kirkham M (2002). 'Use of evidence based leaflets to promote informed choice in maternity care: randomised controlled trial in everyday practice'. *BMJ*, vol 324, p 643.

Okamura K, Bernstein J, Fidler AT (2002). 'Assessing the quality of infertility resources on the World Wide Web: tools to guide clients through the maze of fact and fiction'. *Journal of Midwifery & Women's Health*, vol 47, pp 264–8.

Oliver S, Rajan L, Turner H, Oakley A, Entwistle V, Watt I, Sheldon TA, Rosser J (1996). 'Informed choice for users of health services: views on ultrasonography leaflets of women in early pregnancy, midwives, and ultrasonographers'. *BMJ*, vol 313, pp 1251–55.

Paul F, Cumming P, Fleck E (2001). 'Patient information: involving the user group'. *Professional Nurse*, vol 16, pp 1405–8.

Pearce L (2002). 'A need to know'. *Nursing Standard*, vol 16(43), pp 14–5.

Raynor DK (1998). 'The influence of written information on patient knowledge and adherence to treatment', in *Adherence to Treatment in Medical Conditions*, Myers L, Midence K eds. London: Harwood Academic.

Richardson K, Moran S (1995). 'Developing standards for patient information. Highlights that effective communication can improve health care delivery'. *International Journal of Health Care Quality Assurance*, vol 8, pp 27–31.

Risk A, Dzenowagis J (2001). 'Review of Internet information quality initiatives'. *Journal of Medical Internet Research*, vol 3, p 28.

Salford Centre for Health Promotion (1994). *Getting it Right When You Write*. Salford: SCHP.

Scott C (2001). 'The quality of patient information'. *Professional Nurse*, vol 16, p 1392.

Silver R (1991). *Guidelines: Better information literature for hospital patients*. London: King's Fund.

Smith CE, Cha J, Puno F, Magee JD, Bingham J, Van Gorp M (2002). 'Quality assurance processes for designing patient education web sites'. *Computers, Informatics, Nursing*, vol 20, pp 191–200.

Stapleton H, Kirkham M, Thomas G (2002). 'Qualitative study of evidence based leaflets in maternity care'. *BMJ*, vol 324, p 639.

Strydom A, Hall I (2001). 'Randomized trial of psychotropic medication information leaflets for people with intellectual disability'. *Journal of Intellectual Disability Research*, vol 45, pp 146–51.

Sturdee DW (2000). 'The importance of patient education in improving compliance'. *Climacteric*, vol 3, suppl 2, pp 9–13.

Taylor H (2001). 'The importance of providing good patient information'. *Professional Nurse*, vol 17, pp 34–6.

Terrence Higgins Trust (2002). *Living Well with HIV – A guide to eating well*. London: THT.

Thomas R, Daly M, Perryman B, Stockton D (2000). 'Forewarned is forearmed – benefits of preparatory information on video cassette for patients receiving chemotherapy or radiotherapy – a randomised controlled trial'. *European Journal of Cancer*, vol 36, pp 1536–43.

Thompson S, Stewart K (2001). 'Older persons' opinions about, and sources of, prescription drug information'. *International Journal of Pharmacy Practice*, vol 9, pp 3–162.

Thomson H, Daly M, Perryman B, Stockton D (2002). 'Mothers' use of and attitudes to BabyCheck'. *British Journal of General Practice*, vol 52, pp 314–6.

Welsh S, Anagnostelis B, Cooke A (2001). *Finding and Using Medical Information on the Internet*. London: Aslib-IMI.

Whatley S, Mamdani M, Upshur REG (2002). 'A randomised comparison of the effect of three patient information leaflet models on older patients' treatment intentions'. *British Journal of General Practice*, vol 52, pp 479–84.

White PJ (2002). 'Evidence-based medicine for consumers: a role for the Cochrane Collaboration'. *Journal of the Medical Library Association*, vol 90, pp 218–22.

Wilkinson M, McPherson S (2002). 'NHS Direct Online and the information divide'. *He@lth Information on the Internet*, vol 22, pp 8–10.

Willock J, Grogan S (1998). 'Involving families in the production of patient information literature'. *Professional Nurse*, vol 13, pp 351–4.

Wyatt JC (2000). 'Information for patients'. *Journal of the Royal Society of Medicine*, vol 93, pp 467–71.

Current awareness – keeping up to date

For those wishing to keep abreast of developments in patient information, this section provides a small selection of dedicated publications:

■ *CHIC Update*. Quarterly newsletter produced by the Consumer Health Information Consortium. Tel: 020 7928 9292 x 2507 @ www.omni.ac.uk/CHIC
■ *Patient Information Forum Newsletter*. Available to members of PiF. Email: Mary Last, Editor – mary@waspies.fsnet.co.uk

In addition, a number of journals feature patient information articles. Listed below are some that regularly publish material in this area. Advice on how to identify additional references, and journals, can be found in the Bibliography (*see* p 117).

■ *British Medical Journal* aims to publish rigorous, accessible and entertaining material that will help doctors and medical students in their daily practice, lifelong learning and career development @ www.bmj.com
■ *Health Education Research* deals with issues involved in health education and promotion worldwide – providing a link between the researcher and the results obtained by practising health educators and communicators @ http://her.oupjournals.org
■ *Health Expectations*. An international journal on public participation in health care and health policy @ www.blackwell-science.com/online
■ *Journal of the Royal Society of Medicine* is a leading general medical journal reflecting current thinking and practice across the range of specialties @ www.rsm.ac.uk/pub/jrsm.htm
■ *Nursing Standard* is a leading UK weekly nursing journal @ www.nursing-standard.co.uk
■ *Patient Education and Counseling* is an interdisciplinary, international journal for patient education and health promotion researchers, managers and clinicians @ www.elsevier.com/locate/pateducou
■ *Social Science and Medicine* provides an international and interdisciplinary forum for the dissemination of research findings, reviews and theory in all areas of common interest to social scientists and health practitioners and policy makers @ www.elsevier.com/inca/publications/store/3/1/5/index.htt

Index

Related King's Fund titles

Changing Relationships
FINDINGS OF THE PATIENT INVOLVEMENT PROJECT
Rosemary Gillespie, Dominique Florin and Steve Gillam

Recent years have seen rapid and significant changes in the social, political and policy context of relationships between health professionals and patients. This paper reports on a King's Fund study that reviews the policy framework for patient involvement, and the Government's emphasis on patient-centred health care. It is based on interviews with 45 health care professionals, patient organisations, clinical professional bodies and allied professional groups about how they are taking patient involvement forward in practice.

ISBN 1 85717 468 2   Sept 2002   32 pp   Price £6.00

Every Voice Counts
PRIMARY CARE ORGANISATIONS AND PUBLIC INVOLVEMENT
Will Anderson, Dominique Florin, Stephen Gillam and Lesley Mountford

With primary care trusts (PCTs) now in place nationwide, one of the many challenges they face is to build a greater role for lay people, including patients, carers and communities, in shaping local health and health care services. This publication takes a critical but supportive look at the activities of six London PCTs/PCGs in the period leading up to national implementation, to achieve this goal. It shows that applying national policy to a wide variety of local circumstances to create meaningful public engagement is not easy, but that greater public involvement can bring rich rewards.

ISBN 1 85717 460 7   Mar 2002   90 pp   Price £7.99

Voices, Values and Health
INVOLVING THE PUBLIC IN MORAL DECISIONS
Kristina Staley

Should a congestion charge be introduced in London? Alcohol or drugs programmes: how should a health authority spend its money? This publication reports on a study that asked Londoners to resolve a range of such policy dilemmas. It provides important reading for policy makers and people involved in public values.

ISBN 1 85717 442 9   Jan 2001   58 pp   Price £7.99

New Beginnings
TOWARDS PATIENT AND PUBLIC INVOLVEMENT IN PRIMARY HEALTH CARE
Stephen Gillam and Fiona Brooks (eds)

What matters most for health service users is that they have access to health professionals they can trust. Yet for many decades the health care relationship has been unequal. Doctors have the power and NHS patients should be grateful for what they get. But the balance is changing. This timely book takes up the challenge of effective public involvement and explains how it can add to the value of the NHS.

ISBN 1 85717 439 9   Mar 2001   154 pp   Price £14.99

Health Advocacy for Minority Ethnic Londoners
PUTTING SERVICES ON THE MAP?
Mike Silvera and Rukshana Kapasi

Health advocacy is not an optional extra but an essential tool in improving the health of some of London's most disadvantaged communities, and yet health advocacy remains a marginalised and under-valued activity which is low in status compared to other health and social care professions. This King's Fund publication reports on the findings of the first-ever mapping of the little-understood interface between NHS services and patients from minority ethnic communities, and offers recommendations for improving the service.

ISBN 1 85717 220 5   1998   94 pp   Price £14.99

Involving the Public – One of many priorities
A SURVEY OF PUBLIC INVOLVEMENT IN LONDON'S PRIMARY CARE GROUPS
Will Anderson and Dominique Florin

In what ways, and to what extent, should the public be involved in London's primary care provision? This publication examines the options, including priorities and commitments, resources, leadership, and public involvement to date.

ISBN 1 85717 422 4   May 2000   20 pp   Price £3.00

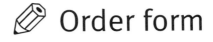 # Order form

Title	ISBN	Price	Quantity
Changing Relationships	1 85717 468 2	£6.00	
Every Voice Counts	1 85717 460 7	£7.99	
Voices, Values and Health	1 85717 442 9	£7.99	
New Beginnings	1 85717 439 9	£14.99	
Health Advocacy for Minority Ethnic Londoners	1 85717 220 5	£14.99	
Involving the Public – One of many priorities	1 85717 422 4	£3.00	

Total £ for titles

Postage and packing

Total order £

☐ I enclose a cheque for £_____
    made payable to King's Fund

☐ Please charge £_____ to my credit card
account   (Please circle: Mastercard/Visa/Visa Delta/Switch)

Card No: _____

Expiry Date: _____

Issue No/Valid from date: _____

Title (Dr, Mr, Ms, Mrs, Miss): _____

First name: _____

Surname: _____

Job title: _____

Organisation: _____

Address: _____

_____

_____ Postcode: _____

Tel: _____ Fax: _____

E-mail: _____

Billing address (if different):

_____

_____

_____ Postcode: _____

POSTAGE AND PACKING – Please add **10%** of the total order value for **UK** (up to a maximum fee of £8.00). Please add **20%** if ordering from **Europe** (up to a maximum of £15.00). Please add **30%** if ordering from the **rest of the world** (up to a maximum of £30.00).

PLEASE NOTE – Shortages must be reported within ten days of delivery date. **We can invoice for orders of £35.00 and over** if a purchase order is supplied.

Please detach and send this order form to:
KING'S FUND
11–13 CAVENDISH SQUARE, LONDON W1G 0AN
TEL **020 7307 2591**   FAX **020 7307 2801**
www.kingsfundbookshop.org.uk

Feedback form

What did you think of *Producing Patient Information: How to research, develop and produce effective information resources*?

Please photocopy this form and return to: *Producing Patient Information* – feedback,
Centre for Health Information Quality (CHIQ), Highcroft, Romsey Road, Winchester, Hampshire SO22 5DH.
Fax: 01962 849 079.

1   Did the guide provide too much, too little or just enough information?

2   Which topics were most useful?

3   Which topics were least useful?

4   What would you wish to see added to or removed from the guide?

5   Did you think the guide was clearly written and presented?

6   Do you think you will use the guide again? If so, how often?

7   Do you produce your own patient information packages?   Yes ☐   No ☐

    If so, have you registered them with the Centre for Health Information Quality (CHIQ)?   Yes ☐   No ☐

8   Any other points?

Name

Position and organisation

Contact details   **Date**